Sticky Blood

explained

by

Kay Thackray

This book is dedicated to Mark Waxman who lost his long fight with this illness but remained strong throughout.

Sticky Blood

explained

Published 2018 by arima publishing

ISBN 978 1 84549 732 3

© Kay Thackray 2018

Printed and bound in the United Kingdom

arima publishing
ASK House, Northgate Avenue
Bury St Edmunds, Suffolk IP32 6BB
t: (+44) 01284 700321

www.arimapublishing.com

Many thanks to the friends and family who have helped me through the years. Special thanks to the Waxman family, Judi Page and Rachel Thackray for their help with editing this book.

Contents

Foreword

The description by Dr Graham Hughes of the "antiphospholipid syndrome" or Hughes Syndrome is one of the medical landmarks of the 20th century.

There is something of a fashion in science to play down 'clinical' discoveries as being somehow less ground-breaking than 'basic' laboratory-based observations.

Here is a disease, a medical discovery, which should turn such fashions around. In a series of brilliant clinical observations, Dr Hughes, not only pieced together what is now clearly a common and important disease, but also, with his team, set up the blood tests and treatment guidelines, which are used worldwide.

In a series of clinical articles in the early 1980s, Dr Hughes and his team described the headaches, the miscarriages, the clotting tendency, the effect on platelets, the strokes, the memory loss... and almost all the clinical picture now recognised as a distinct syndrome.

This was not an anecdotal observation. It was a prime example of meticulous clinical observation and dogged determination. Hughes Syndrome is now recognised as a major 'new' disease. It has been described, by my colleague, Dr Josep Font of Barcelona, as, "one of the 2 new diseases (with AIDS) of the 20th century".

Despite being over 30 years old and being of major importance in the diagnosis of strokes, migraine, multiple sclerosis, and miscarriage, the syndrome is still under diagnosed by doctors.

What about patients? Imagine the 'double insult' of suffering a potentially dangerous (and potentially treatable!) disease, which the doctor has never heard of. In my weekly special pregnancy clinic at St Thomas Hospital, I regularly see patients whose previous symptoms have gone undiagnosed, not to mention their, often multiple, pregnancy losses.

It is for these reasons above all, that I welcome a book such as this.

Kay Thackray has, with this volume, made an important contribution to the understanding of the syndrome.

The messages are simple. Blood clots can cause untold damage. The tendency to 'sticky blood' found in Hughes Syndrome can be diagnosed by simple blood tests. The use of medicines, some as simple as aspirin, can protect against the clotting tendency.

Kay Thackray here provides just the sort of clear guidance patients with Hughes Syndrome need. Coming from a patient, and coming straight from the heart, I believe that the lessons provided by this book are beyond value.

Munther A Khamashta MD FRCP
Consultant Physician, Lupus Unit
ST THOMAS' HOSPITAL, LONDON

Introduction

There is an illness that strikes young people, mainly under 40 years of age.

In that age group it causes, 1 in 5 of all strokes, 1 in 5 of all recurrent miscarriages, also deep vein thrombosis (so-called economy class syndrome), heart attacks, pulmonary embolism (blood clots in the lungs) and in the worst cases amputations or even death.

The list of problems that can be caused by this disease is diverse, from mild to life threatening, from migraines to multiple sclerosis.

Most of us imagine that if an illness, such as this, attacked so many relatively young people, we would have heard of it. Certainly, we think that doctors know all about it and how to treat it.

Sadly, we would be wrong. The truth is that many doctors seem to know little or nothing about what they consider to be a rare disorder.

The illness is Antiphospholipid Syndrome (APS), also named Hughes Syndrome after Professor Graham Hughes, who first described it fully in 1983.

Awareness of the Antiphospholipid Syndrome is very sparse amongst those in the medical profession. As yet only those involved in research seem to be knowledgeable.

Many doctors tend to have vague or outdated ideas about how to treat this syndrome.

I base this observation on my own experience, and that of others, of this serious disorder. This is simply not good enough. It can be deeply distressing to have to deal with doctor after doctor who dismisses your fears and seems to be ill informed, indeed it can also be very dangerous.

There is no one to blame for this lack of awareness, all relatively newly described illnesses go through a period of being poorly understood by doctors and the public, but the balance needs to alter to save lives.

The word needs to spread and heard by the medical profession and the population in general.

If a patient is lucky enough to be diagnosed, which is a feat in itself; the correct treatment is very hard to obtain without considerable determination. Even when APS patients are well informed about what they need to do to prevent further clotting, they may find they have enormous difficulty convincing doctors that they are right.

Without the correct treatment many will go on to suffer multiple clotting incidents until they are disabled or dead. All this in what should be the prime of their life.

This illness is poorly understood worldwide. However, the UK is among the world's leaders concerning research and knowledge about Antiphospholipid Syndrome.

At the London Bridge Hospital in the UK, Professor Hughes and his team of experts are constantly researching this illness and treating those lucky enough to get the holy grail - A REFERRAL!

This is not a rare syndrome but is thought of as such because it is severely under diagnosed and under treated.

It is not difficult to test for Antiphospholipid Syndrome, it's just a blood test - cheap and easy. It is equally as easy to treat it and save people from the permanent disability that a clot may cause.

At present, the treatment comes after you have had a blood clot, which can be too late.

As a person who has been on the receiving end and having spoken to many worldwide in the same situation, I now feel qualified to explain in a friendly and uncomplicated way, to those who are newly diagnosed, exactly what they are up against.

Hopefully my writing will also be of interest to doctors. It is relatively easy to study an illness, reading all about the symptoms is interesting, even fascinating.

Living with Antiphospholipid Syndrome is quite different from researching it or treating people with the disorder.

There are elements of Antiphospholipid Syndrome which have never been written about before; elements which only a fellow patient can truly understand.

I hope that if just a few doctors read this book perhaps they will have a better understanding of the problems faced by people with this syndrome. This book has evolved very slowly as I have learned more from others with Antiphospholipid Syndrome, as each question or problem amongst my many contacts has cropped up, I have added to my writing and tried to find the answers. I hope I have succeeded in finding an answer to your questions.

This is my updated version of the book. I have kept much of it the same as it was back in 2000 as this is my story but have tried to update other parts where new discoveries have changed treatment over the years.

This is written for all survivors of Hughes Syndrome.

Chapter 1

What the heck is Antiphospholipid Syndrome?

This is the question on everybody's lips the first time a doctor tells them they have Antiphospholipid Syndrome. I will attempt to give answers that are a little simplified without leaving anything out that I feel the average patient would be interested in. Firstly, a potted history of the illness is needed. As the name is so cumbersome, and hard to say or spell for most ordinary mortals we will use APS as an acronym for Antiphospholipid Syndrome.

History

APS is also known as Hughes Syndrome, so named after Professor Graham Hughes who was the first to fully describe this syndrome. He was based at St Thomas' Hospital in London until his retirement, however he continues to work on improving the outlook for patients at the London Bridge Hospital with an international team of doctors. In the early 1980s Professor Hughes and his team described the group of clinical features that characterise the Antiphospholipid Syndrome. They found that the tendency for the blood to clot or become 'sticky' was associated with certain antibodies. This discovery led to the standardisation of the blood tests needed to diagnose the syndrome.

At that time a great deal of research took place at the Rayne Institute at St Thomas' Hospital by Professor Hughes and his team. They had the advantage of researching the illness whilst treating actual patients at their clinic. This combination has led to a much better understanding of APS.

APS is an autoimmune disease, which means that instead of your antibodies sticking to attacking flu and measles, they are attacking you. Autoimmunity is medically explained as a condition in which a person's body makes antibodies against its own cells (an antibody is a protein substance made by the body's white blood cells to defend against bacteria and other foreign substances.) There are many types of autoimmune disorders and many of their symptoms are similar; therefore, it is sometimes difficult to diagnose any of these disorders.

In a person with APS, these antibodies attack the blood platelets and cause them to become too sticky and more likely to clot together.

Healthy people have blood that clots, it is necessary for healing wounds, but in APS this mechanism goes into overdrive. Professor Hughes compares the 'sticky' blood to a car engine running on a too rich mix of petrol. It stutters and gets choked up. Since your blood is needed by every area in your body to supply oxygen, APS can affect almost any part of the body, which is why it presents with such strange and varied symptoms.

It is not really known why some people develop autoimmune diseases such as APS. There may be a trigger, such as a virus attack or a shock of some sort and there may also be a hereditary cause. Hormones, whether natural or in tablet form can seem to aggravate sticky blood. Therefore, the contraceptive pill is not recommended for women with Hughes Syndrome. Recently I have read that people who have suffered abuse which has caused their fight or flight hormones to be released far too often over a long period of time seem to have far more likelihood of developing an autoimmune illness. It is an interesting and plausible idea, but more research is needed before anyone can say for sure why autoimmune diseases, such as APS, develop in one person and not another. Stress is obviously also a trigger for most autoimmune illnesses.

Most of those diagnosed with APS are young females. Most of my friends who have APS seem to be in their 30s and 40s and are female, but I also know some as young as their teens and as old as in their 70s or 80s.

It is not confined to women, I have known lots of men with APS through my online work for the illness and sadly not all are still alive today. Men with Hughes Syndrome are outnumbered by women perhaps due to the hormonal changes women experience.

What are the symptoms?

The symptoms are many and varied and may come and go of their own free will. It is unlikely that you will have them all (thank goodness!). You may have one or two of the symptoms one week and different ones the next week. Occasionally you may be lucky and get a break with no symptoms. It is important that you do not panic, just because it's on the list, it doesn't mean you'll develop it!

Some suffer from most of the symptoms on the list and there are others who never really feel ill but developed a clot 'out of the blue' The degree of illness can vary a huge amount between different people.

Likely symptoms are:

• Fuzzy headaches/migraines; sometimes dating back to teenage years, long before diagnosis. These may go on for days at a time and really take over your life, or sometimes just an odd day here or there. These often have limited response to painkillers or migraine medications.

• Pins and needles/numbness; usually in the hands and feet but sometimes elsewhere. It comes on for no reason and can become quite painful or uncomfortable. There may also be hot and cold feelings in the feet or hands, it may feel as though you trod in cold or hot water momentarily.

• Visual disturbances; that can vary from small flashes of light to complicated flickering cog shapes appearing without warning, often in a corner of your vision. This normally lasts for a few minutes, but some people have experienced it for longer.

• Dizziness/Vertigo; Dizziness is a feeling that most of us, with or without this disorder, have encountered. Vertigo is a feeling that the room is spinning or that you may feel that your body is moving and all else is stable. Vertigo can become so severe that you may lose your balance and become so nauseated that vomiting occurs. There is medication to alleviate vertigo. However, when vertigo is due to APS once the blood is thinned this may not be necessary.

- Problems with speech/slurring; sometimes you may use an inappropriate word, or your speech may become slurred. In severe cases, you may speak complete nonsense.

- Co-ordination problems; small things such as doing up buttons or shoes may become more difficult. You may bump into things more often.

- Muscle pain/cramps; these can vary between feeling as though you have run a marathon when you didn't, to severe cramping pain and muscle spasms. You may also notice muscle twitching which may cause your fingers to move involuntarily (or any other affected part of the body.) This usually happens when you are severely fatigued.

- Blurred vision/double vision; your vision may cloud over from time to time, or you may see double, especially when first opening your eyes. Reading and any other close work may become impossible.

- Memory loss; Again, this can be so serious that you forget important things like your address for a moment or mild enough to mean you need to keep a diary to remember your day's appointments. Remembering to take daily medication can be a problem, having routines such as setting out the day's tablets and ticking in a diary when you take them can help if, like me, you are prone to forgetting whether you have taken them.

- Extreme fatigue; this is hard for a normal person to understand. It is not like ordinary tiredness. It is overwhelming and impossible to fight. The smallest task seems impossible when this hits you. The only solution is to rest. It is surprising how refreshed you may feel after a small nap. However, I usually find that once the fatigue sets in, even after a rest, I am inclined to feel tired again far more quickly than anyone else I know! Fatigue can mean you wake up still exhausted after a full night's sleep.

- Livedo Reticularis (blotchy skin); this is a pattern of the blood vessels under the skin resembling tartan! Usually this is seen on the legs. However, it can also occur on the arms, trunk and buttocks. There is usually no treatment. Livedo Reticularis can be permanent or this mottled pattern can come and go on your legs, (or wherever you may have it). It is commonly seen after exposure to sun or cold.

- Brain 'fog'; an inability to think straight. Occasionally you may get lost in the middle of a sentence and completely forget what you were talking about. You may find you have done odd things like putting something away in the wrong place. Sometimes it is a real struggle to keep your mind on the subject in hand; it becomes very easy to be distracted. Saying the wrong word when speaking is common, I have a habit of saying prison instead of hospital!

- Transient Ischemic Attacks (TIAs); a mini stroke, this is described in further detail in a later chapter. This is usually a sign of an impending stroke when pieces of blood clots block an artery leading to the brain so depriving the brain of oxygen. The difference between a TIA and regular stroke is that with a TIA, the artery is usually only blocked for a short time, with a stroke, the blockage lasts longer and causes brain damage. TIAs usually appear suddenly and last less than 24 hours. Symptoms include vision disturbances, fainting or dizziness, a weak or numb feeling on one side of the face or body, or trouble swallowing or speaking.

- Epilepsy; some epileptic patients have been found to have APS. This can often take the form of absences rather than fits but either can be caused by Hughes Syndrome.

- Low platelet count; strangely APS can sometimes cause a lack of blood platelets as well as extreme clotting (a platelet is a blood component responsible for clotting).

- Blood clots almost anywhere in the body; this may cause a stroke, heart attack, pulmonary embolism or thrombosis in the limbs.

Indeed, a clot anywhere in the body that gets lodged and cuts off the blood supply will cause problems.

Blood clots large enough to cut off supply may be surgically removed or injected with a medication known as a "clot buster." However, in most cases, the treatment for blood clots are Heparin or Warfarin therapy to ensure that other clots do not form. Non-life-threatening blood clots may dissolve on their own once the blood is thinned.

- Women may suffer miscarriage, low birth weight babies or pre-eclampsia.

- Splinter haemorrhages; in the finger or toe nails. These appear as bluish lines running from bottom to top of the nail.

- Leg ulcers; often with varicose veins. Varicose veins are swollen veins that you can see under the skin, usually in the legs. These may develop ulcers in severe cases, which may be very difficult to heal.

- Chest pain/angina; which is described in more detail in a later chapter.

- Hearing Loss; you may have a sudden loss of hearing in one or both ears caused by the lack of circulation. A blood clot blocking the supply of blood to the ears can cause deafness within a minute. Sticky blood "clogging things up" in the blood supply to your ears could also cause hearing loss

- Heart valve problems; in severe cases APS can affect the heart valves. This sometimes causes a condition called Libman Sacks Endocarditis, which affects the heart valves and can make them a little leaky. A doctor listening to your heart may hear this problem, as a heart murmur. It is important to stress that this is not a common problem.

- Intermittent claudication; this is a feeling of pain or discomfort, in the leg muscles, often when climbing a slope or steps. It goes away if you rest for a moment and really does just force you to stop. I suppose you could say it feels like the stitch in your side you got as a child when running around for too long, but in your legs instead. It is best to stop, rest and then try again once the pain is gone. "Furred" leg arteries can cause the problem, or sometimes spasms in the leg arteries or just having very sticky blood, any of these will cause poor blood flow. It basically means the leg muscles have insufficient blood flow, for whatever reason, to supply them with the oxygen needed to get you up those steps.

• Metatarsal Bone fracture; the lack of blood supply to the feet can cause bones to weaken and break spontaneously in some patients.

• Angina of the gut; this is caused by the digestive system not having enough oxygen to do its job. It causes abdominal pain after eating.

As the brain is the most sensitive organ to the effects of sticky blood it complains in a variety of ways. These include difficulty with comprehension, concentration, performing calculations, spelling etc and can also include mood swings, anxiety and depression. Anxiety and Depression can be caused by the worry of having the illness but also can be caused by the lack of oxygen supply to certain areas of the brain. Really anything that the brain controls can be affected by a lack of oxygen caused by sticky blood so there will be many more weird symptoms that can be explained by APS.

This is a very long list, but it is important to repeat that you must not panic. You may never experience lots of these symptoms. However, it is important to know them and report them to your doctor if they do.

Indeed, any strange symptoms, even if they are not listed above, should be reported to a doctor.

With treatment, most of these symptoms may either disappear or improve to the extent that they become easier to live with. There is more about treatment in the next chapter.

The main worries with blood clotting are the more serious events such as strokes, heart attacks and thrombosis.

These events are what cause us to be afraid and that is why it is important to be seen by a knowledgeable, up-to-date doctor as soon as possible after diagnosis. Also, you need to find out as much as you can for yourself, don't ever sit back and hope for the best.

Chapter 2

Diagnosis, Treatment and Prognosis

So much for keeping it simple! Basically, this chapter covers:

How do I know I've got it?

What is there I can do about it?

and, most importantly, will I live to see my grandchildren?

Isn't that all we want to know really?!

Diagnosis

The tests and what they are looking for

The tests for APS are called Lupus Anticoagulant, Anticardiolipin Antibodies and Beta-2 Glycoprotein 1 (ß2GP1). Usually full coagulation tests are completed. These check your blood for all blood clotting illnesses and involve taking several small test tubes of blood, so look away if you're nervous. Usually the most important antibodies for clotting on the blood test results are called IgG.

The levels of the IgG antibody in the blood are measured as follows; low positive is between 0 and 15, (if the result is this low you don't necessarily have APS, normal people have some of these antibodies as well sometimes).

medium is between 15 and 50.

high is over 50 units.

However, the antibody levels are not always significant, and a low positive person can be much more ill than a high positive person. The important thing is whether you test positive or not and how you feel. There are other tests for APS, one is the Russell Viper venom test and the other is a false positive for syphilis! I bet that test result has caused some upset in its time! There are also new tests in development.

You don't need to test positive for all three tests, one positive result is all that counts. This is often followed up by a second test a few weeks later to confirm the diagnosis.

Why do people get tested for APS?

Some people discover they have this disease because they have a lot of weird symptoms and an enlightened doctor decides to test for the antibodies.

If this is the case for you, then you are very lucky.

With the correct treatment you may never have a blood clot and some of your nastier symptoms may also disappear.

Sadly, most people, including me, are only tested for the antibodies after a clot has occurred, such as a deep vein thrombosis, a stroke or a heart attack (or, indeed a blood clot anywhere else.) Some people must go through many blood clots before the penny drops and they are finally tested. I have spoken to many, many people on the internet who are permanently disabled now after a couple of strokes or heart attacks.

A simple blood test at the first symptoms could have saved them from disability.

Women are sometimes diagnosed after many miscarriages and with the correct treatment they have gone on to have healthy babies. Strangely, these ladies may never have a problem when they are not pregnant. Since knowledge of this illness is so limited, it isn't really known whether these people will go on to develop APS later. Even if all seems fine, if a person has APS during pregnancy they should know all about the symptoms of sticky blood, and then be vigilant for any worrying signs in the future.

If you have the symptoms described in the last chapter and test positive you need to see a doctor who knows about APS and its implications.

APS with negative blood tests.

There seems to be a small percentage of people (perhaps 5%), who have APS even though their blood tests show nothing. This is very difficult to deal with if you are the patient concerned. Doctors in most local hospitals would scoff at such an idea. Professor Hughes would often treat a person who has classic symptoms and has had blood clots. His view is that the tests are not yet refined enough to pick up every case of APS. If the patient shows the signs of APS and when treated their problems improve, that is probably proof enough that they have APS. In time more tests will be found. Until then at least if these people are treated they are safe. Although Professor Hughes and some of the more knowledgeable doctors have the approach above, don't be surprised if other doctors doubt this theory, minds are often very closed to new developments in every field and medicine is no exception.

Surely all doctors understand Hughes Syndrome, don't they?

Doctors are not gods; there are many excellent practitioners and some not so good ones. Lots of doctors, who may know a lot about other illnesses, know little or nothing about APS and the seriousness of its implications.

Some admit they don't know much about APS and others insist they know even when it is obvious they don't, some really do understand, you must sort out which type you have!

You must speak out if you disagree with what you are told; if the doctor is a good one, he or she should listen and try to help. If he or she is a little pompous you may be wasting your breath, in which case you should seek a second opinion.

Incorrect treatment can be life threatening. I had one doctor who didn't want to treat me until I'd had another clot! He felt I was too young for long-term Warfarin (medication for "blood thinning") even though I'd had a heart attack. If he had been up to date with the current thinking on APS, he would have instantly prescribed life-long Warfarin treatment; because of my symptoms, history of a heart attack and a high positive blood test. I'm sure he meant well but his lack of knowledge of current treatment could have left me disabled or dead!

I chose not to take his advice, but only because I was well informed about the work of Professor Hughes.

Without this knowledge I would have gone blindly on, trusting the doctor, as is the accepted way.

That thought terrifies me. Writing this book is my way of trying to ensure nobody else is put at risk like that. Sadly, I know that at present many people still receive similar advice and worse still, take it!

Treatment

The treatment for this problem is to 'thin' the blood, usually with Warfarin, but sometimes with aspirin or Heparin, or a combination. These medications are often called 'blood thinners' but disable the blood from clotting at the dangerous rate it normally does. You will need to be tested regularly to ensure that the medication is keeping your blood from clotting abnormally, but also to ensure that your blood does not disable clotting too much, as that can cause haemorrhage.

The Grey Area

There is also a grey area of people who test positive for APS but have not had a blood-clotting incident.

If this is you and you have nasty symptoms as previously described there is now a compromise.

Many experts now offer a trial of a few weeks on Heparin injections to see if the symptoms improve at all. The trial is Heparin, rather than Warfarin, as it is easier to control and has less risk of abnormal bleeding. If the Heparin does improve symptoms, then Prof Hughes would recommend long-term Warfarin treatment to protect against future clotting episodes. Warfarin is usually used in the long term rather than Heparin as there is evidence that long-term Heparin can cause osteoporosis! (it's not fair really is it?). In other words, if thinning your blood relieves your symptoms, then the chances are that you would develop a clot sooner or later without thinning your blood. Most of us, when faced with that thought, would say "hand me the Warfarin!" However, the choice is always yours. There are newer treatments to be used in these cases too, as described below.

Clear-Cut APS

If you are a clear-cut case of APS and have had a positive test and a clotting incident to prove it, then you need treatment without any doubt. Few of us would argue with that after a stroke, heart attack, pulmonary embolism or DVT!

Treatments Available

Warfarin

Warfarin is a very safe drug, which has been in use for at least 40 years, so it is well tested and is usually well tolerated. There are side effects in extreme cases, but problems are unusual. It is usually the drug of choice to treat APS and most people manage the regime of tablets and blood tests once they get used to it.

If you are taking Warfarin, you must ask your doctor what INR (international normalized ratio - a measurement of the time it takes for your blood to clot) he or she is aiming for (always above 3).

Warfarin dosing can be a little strange. Weight is not a factor in achieving the correct INR; for instance, a person weighing 7 stone could need more Warfarin than a person weighing 20 stone. One person may take 12 mg of Warfarin daily to get to an INR of 3 and another may only need 5 mg each day. There aren't any rules to tell how large your dose of Warfarin needs to be to reach your target INR.

It can be a sensitive business getting things just right, so you may have odd doses like 5 mg daily and 6 mg on a Sunday! Your blood will be tested daily until it is at the correct INR and stable.

After that you may get away with weekly, bi-weekly or monthly checks. The side effects are few, mainly bruising and more rarely slight hair thinning in some people. You will need several packets of tablets as they come in different doses (you may have about 4 boxes of tablets in the different doses such as 0.5mg, lmg, 3mg, 5mg, to use to make up the dose your anticoagulation clinic tells you to take). It is vital to take your

Warfarin at roughly the same time every day. If you miss a dose never take two doses at once as this can be very dangerous.

About your INR

You may have trouble convincing your local doctor at the anticoagulation clinic to keep your INR high enough, this is because they fear you will haemorrhage, which can be minor, but on very rare occasions, more serious.

It is, therefore, very important to be determined and not let any doctor tell you that a lower INR than you have been told to try for, is acceptable.

It is as well to keep your nerve here. I have read the statistics. There is 10 times more chance of a clot occurring if your Warfarin is low dose, than there is chance of a serious haemorrhage if your blood INR is kept at 3 or a little above.

In other words, it is best to keep the INR high enough to avoid clots, as haemorrhaging is far less likely at an INR of 3 than clots are at an INR of 2.

I realise all of this sounds like a balancing act, but as a rule of thumb if your INR is higher than 3, clotting is unlikely but not impossible.

In this imperfect world all we can do is strive for what is best. Remember as Prof Hughes says, "this is a clotting illness not a bleeding illness".

Your part of the bargain is to take your tablets regularly and try to be constant in your habits. All things in moderation is the best way.

Your INR can fluctuate quite a lot. It can be affected by so many seemingly innocuous things!

Try not to get paranoid about it, just do your best to eat and drink without bingeing or dieting. Also, don't take any weird or wonderful herbal remedies until you have checked with your anticoagulation clinic. The main problem with so many of the so-called 'natural' remedies is that the amounts of active ingredients in each tablet can vary a lot. Your INR can be affected by almost anything you take in tablet form 'natural' or prescribed, or, indeed, 'over the counter'. Pharmacists should be able to tell you what pain killers/flu remedies, etc. are safe to take whilst taking

Warfarin. Make it a rule not to take anything like that without checking with a pharmacist or a doctor whether your INR will be affected.

It is important to remember that some of this is beyond your control and go with the flow; accept it as part of the illness. It will usually settle eventually and, if it doesn't, then try not to become obsessed.

Home INR Testing Kits

Some people with APS have problems controlling their INR. It can swing wildly and so increase the danger of having blood clots, despite taking Warfarin. Unless you are relatively stable the Warfarin clinics tend not to test often enough to keep the INR in the correct range for some people with APS.

Also, it must be said that sitting in a clinic for a couple of hours with elderly and frail people is a little depressing when you are young. Most people taking Warfarin are of retiring age (most of these patients do not have APS or other autoimmune or blood disorders but have had a singular clotting episode and are taking the drug to ensure that no others occur) and, whilst there is nothing wrong with that, it can feel as though you are now bracketed with the older generation! I used to read retirement magazines and feel as though I should at least appear to struggle a little when it was my turn to get up!

If you feel you have had enough of drowning in a sea of elderly folks, or you are afraid to leave the control of your INR to someone else, then it is worthwhile obtaining an INR test kit for home testing. It is also very inconvenient when you are a busy person to have to sit and wait in a clinic for a couple of hours every fortnight. The INR home testing machine works in a very similar way to a blood glucose monitor used by diabetics. This machine gives you the opportunity to test yourself, perhaps weekly or fortnightly depending on how often you need to test your INR.

You can then decide to very slightly up or down the dose of Warfarin, depending on your target INR. The important word being 'slightly', if you have been going to a Warfarin clinic you should know that they usually only alter the dose by a tiny amount at a time.

If you feel uncomfortable about this perhaps a talk with your GP, primary care doctor or consultant will make you feel more confident.

It is not a step to take lightly but some people will find this method is their saviour. After all, if you get a scary reading and feel it would be better to have some supervision you can always go back to your clinic until your INR settles down. A good, understanding GP/ primary care doctor is a real godsend as well. You can always arrange to test yourself and then report to the clinic for advice on altering your dose if you are nervous about self-medicating. Also many clinics will allow you to test your own blood and report the result to them so that they can advise on dosage, this may be a good plan if you are not confident enough to decide on your own dose.

The downside is that the machines are quite costly and not available on the NHS (National Health Service in the UK, although the test strips are now available through the NHS) or through most medical insurances in the US. Compared to the risk of blood clots, many of us would feel the cost of the machine is a price worth paying.

The treatment is life-long so never let a doctor tell you to discontinue taking Warfarin unless you are positive they know what they are talking about. Even if your antibodies disappear, which they can do, the risk of clots is much worse than any problems taking Warfarin.

Play it safe "just keep taking the tablets!"

What if I my blood gets "too" thin'?

Do be vigilant, and report things like recurrent nosebleeds, blood in your urine or stools, or bleeding of any sort that seems abnormal. But, don't panic - often it is not anything at all to do with the Warfarin.

Just be sure and get it checked out. Just because your blood is 'thinner' than normal it doesn't mean you won't be able to stop bleeding. If your INR is in range you may take a little longer to stop bleeding if you cut yourself, that is all.

If any part of your body bleeds for more than 15 minutes go to hospital, even if it seems ok. Take care, be over cautious, and always keep a record of your INR readings with you. Never be afraid to make a fuss about getting your INR checked if you feel it is necessary. It is your body and your blood and you must try to be in control as much as you can.

In case of a serious bleed or an accident you will often be given an injection of Vitamin K. Vitamin K counteracts the 'blood thinning' effects of Warfarin.

For this reason, whilst taking Warfarin it is advisable not to take any vitamin tablets containing Vitamin K.

It is also reasonable if you have trouble maintaining your target INR to look at the amount of Vitamin K in your diet. Green leafy vegetables often have lots of Vitamin K and whilst they shouldn't be avoided unless you really are having a terrible time with your INR, it is a good idea to stay constant in the amount of Vitamin K rich foods you eat.

I don't mean measuring anything or cutting anything out of your diet. I'm just saying, don't eat ten helpings of broccoli one day and then none for the rest of the week, try to be constant.

Vitamin K is also found in fat substitutes, such as Olestra, and certain vegetable oils.

When in hospital I would never allow anyone to give me Vitamin K unless I was bleeding to death. It can really be dangerous to have your INR drop to 1 very suddenly. Emergency use only is my rule.

Heparin

Heparin is often used in place of Warfarin in the cases of pregnancy (as Warfarin can cause birth defects) or for those who cannot tolerate Warfarin and those who find it hard to maintain their INR.

This involves injecting yourself, which sounds awful, but really doesn't hurt too much.

A low molecular weight Heparin is often used, as it is less likely to cause osteoporosis when used long-term. You should ask your doctor about this.

Your doctor will advise you on dosage and testing your blood. You should also be shown how to inject yourself. The dose of Heparin is decided based on your body weight. This means it is more controllable and predictable than Warfarin and doesn't need regular blood tests in the same way.

Heparin is soon removed from your system, unlike Warfarin, which can take a few days. For this reason, Heparin is often used when surgery is needed and then you may switch back to Warfarin afterwards. This is known as bridging.

I don't often need Heparin unless my INR is below 3 or I need to stop Warfarin for a medical procedure, but there are a few tips from women with experience in these matters. One is not to rub where you have injected as it makes the bruising worse. Do not bathe or shower 10 minutes before or after injecting for the same reason. Also, and this is common sense, try to vary the site that you inject to avoid getting too sore in one place. The usual place to inject yourself is in the stomach or anywhere quite fleshy (this is one of those times when a little blubber can be useful!) If using the stomach, try not to inject too close to the navel as I am reliably informed the bruising is worse. Arnica cream or a cold compress will help.

Injecting yourself is not a pleasant thing to have to do, but for most determined would be mothers, it is a small price to pay for a successful pregnancy.

After all, it is no more than diabetics do all their lives.

Aspirin

Aspirin alone may be used for mild cases of APS, or with Warfarin or Heparin, for either more severe cases or in pregnancy. Some people may tell you that aspirin and Warfarin cannot be taken together, but in the case of APS it is fine if your doctor advises it.

The tablets are not the same as those you buy for a headache. They are low dose 'baby' aspirin, usually 75mg. The worst side effect of long-term aspirin therapy can be stomach ulcers. To protect yourself against such ulcers, take coated tablets and always take them after a meal so your stomach is full of food. Apart from this, you should be fine.

Aspirin is already used widely in heart and stroke patients to make the blood less 'sticky' with few problems.

There is an alternative to aspirin, ask your doctor, it is called Plavix (Clopidogrel Bisulphate.) This is an anti-platelet tablet, which has a similar effect to aspirin. It is sometimes used in its place and does not irritate the stomach, your doctor will be able to tell you more.

Hydroxychloroquine

This is sometimes used to treat Lupus.

It is an anti-malarial medication that has been found, coincidentally, to help rheumatic diseases.

Many people with APS also have some of the symptoms of Lupus. Some have full-blown Lupus and others a mild version or just occasional symptoms such as joint pain, which cannot be strictly classified.

Hydroxychloroquine can prevent damage being caused by the illness to organs, joints etc. It can reduce pain and fatigue in some people. A good APS doctor will know when this drug is needed.

As always, doctors must weigh up the pros and cons of using a medication for your symptoms. Hydroxychloroquine is one to discuss with a doctor if you feel it will help you. It can have some unpleasant side effects, but many people find it is a wonderful help and have no side effects. It is up to the individual to decide with the help of his or her doctor whether it might be worth trying.

Newer Anti-Clotting medications

Newer types of anticoagulants are also available and are becoming increasingly common. These include:

Rivaroxaban (Xarelto), Dabigatran. (Pradaxa) and Apixaban (Eliquis).

These are in tablet form and are often now used in people with symptoms but no clots. There are trials into how effective they are for APS patients.

I know of quite a few people taking these drugs, so far successfully. I would advise sticking with tried and tested Warfarin or Heparin however for most of us. In time I believe these newer anticoagulants may be used more as there is no INR testing involved. For now however I prefer not to be a human guinea pig as Warfarin works so well for me.

It is very good though that there is another alternative for those who don't do well on traditional treatments.

Prognosis

If you are careful and take your medications, there is no reason you shouldn't live to be old. This illness needs to be taken seriously as it can be so disabling if patients or doctors do not. I have had this illness for 20 years now, I have grandchildren, I am fitter than I was in my 30s. I have taken good care of myself during this time and that is important.

The best news is that with careful treatment and monitoring we can live a relatively normal life span.

Most of us will manage a reasonably full life. Some of us may be fitter than others, and of course there can still be blips in the treatment but, with care, just about everyone with APS can survive to old age and, more importantly, want to!

There is no reason why you should not see your grandchildren, I have managed to see mine. My next goal is great grandchildren!

Chapter 3

The connection with other diseases

It is an unfair aspect of these auto-immune diseases that often they don't like to stay on their own! It's as if one of them comes to stay and then invites others to join the party (in your body!). As with everything else, if you have APS alone it doesn't mean anything else will develop. It is just as well to know that it is possible however.

Lupus

Some people with Lupus (a miserable deal without anything else), develop APS. This is known as secondary APS.

However, if you have APS first, it is very unusual to develop lupus. If you have APS without lupus it is called primary APS.

Lupus usually refers to Systemic Lupus Erythematosus or SLE for short. It is another autoimmune disease. Lupus's attack on our body can cause inflammation to our tissues.

Most people with Lupus have sore swollen joints and skin rashes. The most well-known rash is the facial one in the shape of a butterfly across the nose and cheeks.

Other symptoms may include sensitivity to the sun, and swollen glands. Fever, extreme fatigue, unusual hair loss, swelling in legs or around the eyes are common symptoms. These symptoms can change dramatically from day to day. In most cases, they disappear for a while, then resurface in bouts called flares. Eventually damage can be caused to the various body tissues affected.

Lupus can be successfully treated and though at one time it was thought to be a death sentence, that is no longer true. There are many books describing Lupus and its treatment etc, so I won't go into any detail.

The test for Lupus is anti-nuclear antibodies. If these are raised, along with the various symptoms, it usually leads to a diagnosis. It is however possible to have Lupus without a positive test if you have most of the symptoms.

The other type of Lupus is Discoid Lupus, which mainly affects the skin with unsightly disc shaped patches of scaly skin. It is relatively unusual for this to be as serious as SLE however as in most cases it is confined to the skin. It can be very disfiguring though, especially if it affects the face.

Thyroid problems

Some people have thyroid troubles, either over or under active. Sometimes this can also be autoimmune.

An over active thyroid causes sweating, weight loss, palpitations, trembling and a feeling of always being hot. The body goes into complete overdrive making everything work much faster and increasing your metabolism.

An under active thyroid has the opposite effect, slowing the body down. The metabolism slows, causing sensitivity to the cold, weight gain, tiredness, a slow heartbeat and sometimes depression.

Both problems are easily treated with tablets. Sometimes radioactive treatment or surgery for an overactive thyroid is needed if the tablets are ineffective.

Sjogren's Syndrome

Sjogren's is yet another autoimmune illness, which this time attacks the 'moisture making' glands of the body. This will cause dry mouth, dry gritty eyes, dry skin and joint problems. In women, it also causes you to become 'dry where a girl shouldn't be!' if you get my drift!

The treatment is to replace the moisture with eye drops, drinking a lot, skin creams, and for the more personal problems there are of course gels that are available from any high street pharmacy. Unless the problem is very severe, it is really a case of just moisturise everywhere!

You may have trouble wearing eye makeup as it irritates your eyes. Some brands may be fine and there are many made especially for sensitive skin. You may find your eyes are irritated by bright light, sunlight, strong smells, a blast of heat when opening an oven door can make your eyes momentarily stick together. Always wear sunglasses on a sunny day, remember to stand back when you open the oven, open windows, avoid cigarette smoke if it affects you. Sometimes these irritants will not bother you, other times even though you have dry eyes normally, your eyes will stream because they get very irritated. Get into the habit of carrying a tissue or hanky, people may think you are tearful, just say you have sensitive eyes.

Swallowing dry food can be a trial as well.

Always have a drink with your meals. Some people carry a bottle of water around with them, as a dry mouth can be uncomfortable if you speak for very long. Sugar free gum is useful as it encourages the salivary glands to work and helps to keep the teeth clean. Tooth decay can be a major problem if you have Sjogren's and dental hygiene is very important. You should tell your dentist that you have Sjogren's and then if it causes you problems you can get help. Your skin may get very dry and scaly unless you endlessly moisturise it. Pay special attention to your feet and make sure they get plenty of attention, sore, dry, cracked feet are very painful and to be avoided if you can.

The associated joint pain with Sjogren's is usually something that comes and goes and isn't usually too severe. There are medications to help, so don't be afraid to ask your doctor for help if it gets too painful.

Raynaud's Syndrome

Raynaud's appears as a blueness from lack of circulation to the extremities, usually the fingers and toes. The extremities usually turn pale, then blue and, finally, red. Raynaud's affects most APS patients when their extremities are subject to cold weather. When the small arteries that bring blood to the fingers and toes are exposed to cold, they spasm and contract, reducing the blood supply.

Those who suffer from Raynaud's should be extra cautious to wear warm gloves and socks in the cold seasons. Raynaud's can be painful. Smoking and stress also complicates this syndrome.

Multiple Sclerosis

Multiple Sclerosis (MS) and APS can easily be mistaken for each other. My GP's initial thought (before a scan showed otherwise) was MS. The nervous system is affected by both illnesses and so some of the very odd symptoms are common to both. In fact, when you read a list of MS symptoms most of them apply to untreated APS patients.

Prof Hughes has been testing some MS sufferers for the antibodies connected with APS and had some very interesting results. Since even MRI scans can show similar results for both illnesses, it is down to whether you have the antibodies or have had a clot.

APS is a better diagnosis than MS as, at least, it is more treatable and, in the long-term, usually less disabling. It is important to get the diagnosis correct as untreated APS may lead to a potentially serious blood clot. Also, some very distressing MS symptoms may disappear or at the very least improve when a misdiagnosed person is anticoagulated.

The illnesses can both look the same on an MRI scan of the brain. The "lesions" of Hughes syndrome however can move about like clouds across the sky. The MS lesions stay fixed. If there is any doubt then perhaps two MRI scans should be done with a few months interval to see if the lesions have moved.

To make matter worse APS can affect the myelin sheath around the nerves sometimes. Differentiating between the two is very difficult but a blood clot is not an MS symptom.

If you have had a blood clot it seems very likely that Hughes Syndrome is your problem rather than Multiple Sclerosis.

Cardiac Syndrome X/Microvascular Angina/Prinzmetals

I, along with others, have a type of angina, which is sometimes found with APS. This type of angina is present in people with completely clear coronary arteries, rather than with the clogged ones that are usually the case in the usual form of angina. It is assumed that the chest pain and breathlessness are caused by the coronary arteries contracting of their own accord and restricting the flow of blood to the heart muscle. At other times the arteries may look completely normal on an angiogram. This type of angina is Cardiac Syndrome X or sometimes it gets called Prinzmetals. There is also research to say that Microvascular angina is another cause of angina with clear arteries, as in Microvascular angina the smaller blood vessels are not performing properly, they may spasm or just not function well enough.

It is usually treated with varying success using angina medication and various other drugs to control the attacks. Every case seems to be a little different and trial and error is normally required to find which treatment works. There is no operation for this condition, as there is no blockage to clear.

In my case, the angina is controlled most of the time with a nitrate spray and artery widening tablets. When it gets worse I may need to go to hospital for a few days or put myself on bed rest at home, but I know it is doing my heart no long-term damage if I avoid clots by taking Warfarin.

The use of Warfarin has certainly reduced the seriousness of my angina attacks and has made the onset of angina for me far more predictable than it was before. I have also found that my nitrate spray is now more effective.

Not everyone with Cardiac Syndrome X, or normal angina caused by furred up arteries, will show the same improvement following treatment with Warfarin but if the INR is high enough it should help.

Quite aside from the improvement in the actual angina pain, it is vital that if your arteries are prone to contracting, your blood is not also prone to clotting. That could be a lethal combination! Thank goodness for Warfarin! When I read that people with Cardiac Syndrome X don't usually have heart attacks I shake my head. Try mixing it with APS!

High Blood Pressure

High blood pressure is a nuisance but once again just another tablet can bring it under control, so it's not worth getting too upset. Half the world seems to take blood pressure tablets! If you want to help yourself eat a low-fat diet with as little salt as you can bear and exercise every day you will be able to manage it.

I don't mean a 5-mile jog; just a half-hour striding out is enough. There's no need to get fanatical about any of the advice. In time blood pressure can settle, so it is worth discussing with your doctor the chances of trying to manage without blood pressure tablets some time in the future.

Tummy Troubles

With many tablets to take you may have an irritated acid stomach but guess what? There's a tablet for that, too! Where would we be without them? These reduce the acid in your stomach preventing acid reflux.

If you take aspirin make sure they are the coated type, which are better for your stomach. An irritated stomach can bring on a feeling of pressure from below your stomach, (a bit like being pregnant) it's a bloated feeling that can also make your breathing a little uncomfortable with the 'full' feeling. If there is too much stomach trouble aspirin will be discontinued, as it is well known as an irritant.

Chronic Fatigue Syndrome and Fibromyalgia

Some research has been undertaken into whether some cases of Chronic Fatigue Syndrome are suffering from APS. It would seem logical given that the symptoms are similar. Chronic Fatigue Syndrome has a list of symptoms that sound very similar to many of those felt by APS patients, especially prior to treatment. It seems likely that some of those people may have APS.

Many APS sufferers also have extensive muscle pain at times so Fibromyalgia is another recently talked about illness that may be connected to APS.

Fibromyalgia is a complaint that has only recently been recognized; fibro means muscle and myalgia means pain. If people have other suspicious symptoms as well, testing some of them for APS would perhaps be an interesting idea.

There are so many other connected diseases...

Other connected problems are weird and wonderful, rare and often autoimmune things such as, Scleroderma, Budd-Chiari Syndrome, and Haemolytic Anaemia, basically, anything that is autoimmune is possibly linked to APS. Many people have diabetes with their APS, so could APS have some effect on the pancreas?

Since there are around 80 or more different autoimmune illnesses I won't go into detail about them all, that would be a whole new book! I have tried to mention the most common ones amongst people who have APS.

Weight Control

Many of us also seem to have a problem with weight control as well. Whether this is due to changes in the way our body is working or whether it is due to a reduction in the amount of exercise we can participate in, is not really proved. It does seem however that many people with APS also have weight control difficulties, so it seems likely that in some people changes occur. Really all you can do is try not to worry about what cannot be changed, but also do your best to eat sensibly and exercise when possible.

Do I have lots of illnesses or is it all APS?

It is often hard to say whether the symptoms of other illnesses are just very similar to APS or whether a person is genuinely suffering from two or more illnesses at once.

My personal view is that if it all started together it is unlikely that two separate illnesses attacked at the same time, so most of my strange occurrences I believe are APS.

I do know that other sufferers do have more than one autoimmune illness linked together though and having one autoimmune illness seems to pre-dispose you to developing others. The divisions between the symptoms of various autoimmune illnesses are blurred; you can have mild lupus with APS, or slightly dry eyes, or a strange rash, without having another full-blown illness. It is quite usual to have APS along with a good few nondescript, vague, extra symptoms, which may come and go. If they are mild and not too troublesome usually you can safely ignore them as much as you can.

There are 3 illnesses that Prof Hughes calls the big 3. These are Sjogren's, Hughes syndrome and thyroid problems. Many of us have all 3 together.

It is also possible to just have a cold or flu if you suffer from APS, and for that to make everything seem worse. I always have the flu 'jab' and would recommend anyone with a long-term illness to have it and for pneumonia. We have enough to deal with, who needs anything else! I'm sure there are other connected problems so I'm sorry if I missed yours.

All parties have gatecrashers after all! So sorry if I forgot the invite.

Anxiety about medication

Try not to be anxious about taking tablets for your various illnesses. I swallow mine then forget them.

I never look at the side effects on the leaflet, as if I don't read it I probably won't develop it. Amateur psychology but it often works for me! Study all those leaflets if you are the type that needs to know. We're all different after all.

Please remember if APS is your only problem you must not imagine there is another problem around the corner. Deal with what is happening now, not what may never happen. Just be aware of the possibility and put it to the back of your mind.

Chapter 4

Pregnancy and APS

This is a subject I don't know much about from a personal viewpoint, as I was lucky enough to be unscathed during pregnancy. I only had pre-eclampsia at the end of my first pregnancy, and one emergency caesarean at 34 weeks due to pre-eclampsia, which is nothing compared to the experiences of other women. Pre-eclampsia is a condition in pregnancy that can result from having APS.

What is puzzling about cases with APS and pregnancy is that sometimes women will have health problems when pregnant, including having recurrent miscarriages; however, they may otherwise have no symptoms of APS. This may be because the hormones that flow through the body when pregnant are different from those normally found in the blood stream and these can initiate the APS symptoms.

Others are not so lucky and go on to develop full-blown Hughes Syndrome after pregnancy or even years later. Why this is, no one knows yet.

Perhaps vigilance is the only real answer, to be aware of the symptoms of Hughes Syndrome and report anything odd straight away, even if you have been told that APS will only affect you during pregnancy.

Maybe everyone develops Hughes Syndrome eventually if they are prone to it in pregnancy? No one will really know the answers until more time goes by and more long-term research is done.

Basically, the cause of pregnancy problems with APS patients is that small clots reduce or even cut off the blood supply to the placenta, thus starving the baby of oxygen and nutrition.

In a mild case, the only sign that this is happening is a baby that is not growing sufficiently and is described as small for that stage in the pregnancy. It should have been a 9lb baby but is perhaps a tiny 5lb baby instead, despite being full term.

A more formal name for this is Intra Uterine Growth Retardation (IUGR). Some babies suffering from this at birth, like my first born, grow perfectly normally and to a normal height (my son is now around 6 foot). Others will always be small, or only catch up a little with their peers, usually this happens if the child is short for the amount of weeks of the pregnancy at birth.

If the problem is worse, then pre-eclampsia may set in towards the end of the pregnancy. This causes high blood pressure, protein in the urine and swelling, often of the fingers and ankles, for the mother. For the baby it means that there is a lack of sufficient food and oxygen from the placenta. If severe this usually ends in an early delivery and mother and baby are both at risk whilst blood pressures are soaring. Occasionally, this can end in miscarriage or even a planned abortion to save the mother's life. Pre-eclampsia is most dangerous as it can develop into Eclampsia, which threatens both the mother and the babies' life.

Eclampsia is from the Greek meaning 'bolt from the blue'. It causes the mother to develop seizures and/or decreased consciousness because of untreated or poorly controlled pre-eclampsia.

Another complication of pre-eclampsia is HELLP Syndrome. This syndrome describes a group of symptoms that can occur together in pregnant women. Haemolytic Anaemia (H), elevated liver enzymes (EL), and low platelet count (LP). As this can be very dangerous for both mother and baby, the only treatment is as for Eclampsia, delivery of the baby, no matter how far along in the pregnancy the mother is.

Probably the most distressing problem in pregnancy is the recurrent miscarriage. Often these miscarriages can be well into the pregnancy causing terrible distress. Some are even stillbirths at full-term, which is a dreadful trauma for all concerned. Every mother can understand that a late miscarriage is devastating. By the time this happens the baby has often begun to move, and the mother has already formed a relationship with the life within her. Losing a child at the last moment must be impossible to forget.

Every time this poor mother conceives she is destined to a sad ending and, all too often, she goes through this time after time before anyone will test her for the Hughes Syndrome antibodies. Even then there is no guarantee that she will get expert help unless she is knowledgeable and determined.

Miscarriage is a traumatic experience for a woman and is too often dismissed. However, it takes a very resilient person not to despair after many such losses. Perhaps all women should be given a blood test for the antibodies when they miscarry for the first time. I can see no benefit in prolonging the agony if Hughes Syndrome is the cause.

The treatment for recurrent miscarriage is to thin the blood.

Warfarin cannot be used, as it is known to cause birth defects.

Usually a combination of Heparin and aspirin is used throughout pregnancy, and then discontinued just before a planned delivery.

Heparin injected into the stomach is a daily, uncomfortable experience, but a woman will endure much more than that when she desperately wants a healthy baby.

In some very severe cases, despite all best efforts, it is still very difficult to prevent miscarriages occurring or even sadder, stillbirths.

Most women will persevere, however and with the correct treatment most will go on to give birth to a healthy child eventually. There are many women worldwide who have Hughes Syndrome and have produced healthy offspring so there is a great deal of hope for anyone with the correct treatment. The odds of a healthy baby with treatment are around 80 percent compared to 19 percent without treatment.

The trauma of all this cannot be over emphasised.

It is enough to tip many women over the edge and it can destroy a marriage. It says a lot for the strength of women that they can go through so much and keep trying.

After delivery, some women will be completely fine until they become pregnant again. Others may develop blood clots elsewhere in the body or symptoms of 'sticky' blood and need life-long anticoagulation with Warfarin. As already mentioned, at present there is no way of knowing which women will be fine, and which will not.

It cannot be stressed enough that it is vitally important for all pregnant women who have the antibodies, and a history of problems with miscarriage, to be treated by a knowledgeable doctor at a large teaching hospital that has the required support systems in place.

Expert antenatal care makes all the difference between a sad and happy ending, and no woman should be denied the chance of a successful pregnancy.

Problems with 'that' time of the month!

As it won't be enough to make a whole chapter alone I thought it worth mentioning that one of the side effects of having thinner blood is that your periods can become very heavy and prolonged. Many friends have taken the drastic step of having a hysterectomy and so have I.

My thoughts are that even if you have no desire to add to your family an operation is a bit of a daunting prospect. There are other treatment options to discuss such as endometrial ablation or trying a Mirena IUD first.

If all else fails however and hysterectomy is the answer, then ask about a vaginal hysterectomy. This is far easier to get over as there is no wound across the belly area. It is keyhole surgery and I found it quick to recover from.

Chapter 5

How do I tell...?

This chapter is asking the question most of us need answering from time to time when we're afraid and unsure.

How do I tell if I'm having a stroke or heart attack, DVT, Pulmonary Embolism or TIA?

These are the major blood clotting problems and I will describe the symptoms of each below.

TIA's and Strokes

A TIA (Transient Ischaemic Attack) is often called a mini-stroke. It is called this because recovery is complete and nearly always within 24 hours or even minutes. Symptoms are:

* Brief attacks of numbness, and pins and needles of the face, arm or leg on one side of the body.

* Loss of vision in one eye.

* Slurring of speech or difficulty finding words.

* Sometimes a momentary loss of awareness or surroundings.

These don't usually cause permanent damage but are a sign that all is not well, and you are at increased risk of a stroke. Contact your doctor about this urgently.

The most common signs of Stroke are:

* Sudden numbness or weakness of face, arm or leg on one side of the body.

* Sudden confusion, trouble speaking or understanding.

* Sudden trouble seeing in one or both eyes.

* Sudden trouble walking, dizziness, loss of balance or co-ordination.

* Sudden severe headache with no known cause.

Less common symptoms are:
* Sudden nausea, fever and vomiting that comes on within minutes.

- Brief loss of consciousness or decreased consciousness.

Contact the emergency services immediately if you believe you are having a stroke.

Angina and Heart Attacks

Angina does not usually bring about extreme agony, it is more of a dull ache with a feeling of heaviness and pressure. It is usually felt in the chest, it can also be pain in the back between the shoulders and in the upper arms. This is often accompanied by shortness of breath. It feels like indigestion that will not go away and gets worse and worse unless you sit down and rest. Some describe the pressure as feeling as though an elephant were sitting on your chest.

Angina usually settles with rest and medication within a few minutes, at most half an hour. Exercise, cold, extreme heat or stress usually bring it on. In most cases, your GP will be able to deal with it.

A heart attack may not be painful initially, but usually it becomes very painful as it continues.

Unlike angina you could be doing anything when it strikes, even be asleep!

The symptoms are the same as angina but often feeling much more severe and with a sense of impending doom. You may sweat and look pale.

The pain and pressure do not go away with rest but just keep on and on.

If you suspect you have had a heart attack get emergency help immediately. Don't do what I did and drive yourself to the doctors, get them to come to you or call an ambulance. A heart attack is not always the complete agony that people imagine, but usually you will have a good idea that something serious is happening, and so will those around you.

Early treatment can make a huge difference to survival.

Phlebitis and Deep Vein Thrombosis

Phlebitis is when blood clots form in the veins we can see on the surface (as in varicose veins) you will feel a tender area on the surface of the affected limb, which is swollen. Phlebitis is not dangerous but consult your doctor as soon as possible, they may give you a support bandage to wear.

A deep vein thrombosis is when a clot forms in the deep veins within the affected limb. The limb swells over a period of hours and becomes very painful. You need to see a doctor urgently as a deep vein thrombosis can lead to a Pulmonary Embolism as the blood clot breaks up or moves.

However, you may not have such severe symptoms of swelling and pain. You could feel as if you have pulled a muscle. It is most important to remember to take it seriously if you are having prolonged pain that you have never experienced before, anywhere in your body, and to contact your physician as soon as possible.

Pulmonary Embolism (Blood clot in the lungs)

The symptoms are as follows:

- Chest pain.
- Chronic cough sometimes with blood streaks.
- Difficulty breathing.
- Sweating.
- Shock.
- Bluish skin.
- Anxiety.
- Loss of consciousness.

You need to go to hospital if you suspect that you have a blood clot in your lungs. Seek medical help immediately. These symptoms may not appear all at one time. You may notice that, over time, you cannot perform the daily activities that you normally would without becoming short of breath. Or, you may have chest pain when you take deep breaths, whereas you never had that problem before. The key point to remember is that any new pain or symptom can be a signal of a clot. It could be as severe as going into shock or could be as minor as losing your breath running upstairs.

Thrombocytopenia (low blood platelets)

It is a weird aspect of this illness that it is possible to bleed as well as clot. What did we do to deserve this?

The main symptoms to watch for are:

- Bleeding gums
- Nose bleeds
- Petechiae - small red or purple dots on the skin, often the legs or mouth
- Bruising for no reason
- Fatigue

These symptoms can also be caused by the Warfarin. However, if an excess of any of them worries you, only a blood test can tell whether the platelet count is low. This is a serious problem, not to taken lightly as it is difficult to treat a patient who is bleeding and clotting at the same time! Try not to worry too much, there are drugs to control this condition, and what's another tablet? It may be difficult to treat but it is not at all impossible, I know of lots of people who have come through such an episode and been fine.

Most of us will never know what it is to have this problem, so unless you do, don't waste time worrying over something that may never happen to you.

OK, admit it, now you're afraid

Now I know all this sounds scary, but it is better to know how these things feel so that you have more idea about when to raise the alarm. Not knowing won't prevent anything happening any more than knowing will make anything happen. It is better to panic a little, perhaps needlessly, now and then, than be blasé about APS and bury your head in the sand.

If you are in doubt, play it safe. It is much better to look foolish and to fuss too much than end up disabled or six feet under!

It's hard work living with this illness and having to know about the scary stuff, but the alternative doesn't sound much fun either! So, take care and be vigilant and knowledgeable, but don't go losing sleep worrying about it unless it happens!

Chapter 6

My Own Story

My problems began slowly with the odd vertigo attack, strangely only when I had been asleep. I would wake with a start; the room would be spinning violently, and I would feel I had to be sick.

It would take a few days to recover from but then I would forget all about it until the next time. This would happen every few months and was blamed on the heat, the cold, a virus etc.

It built up until I had headaches. I'd had migraines since I was 14 which is a pointer for APS.

Then there was blurred and double vision, visual disturbances, muscle pain, fatigue, pins and needles and numbness. Also, a dull ache between my shoulder blades whenever I was tired (I now know this as angina). My GP gave me a migraine remedy to try for a month. I can honestly say it made not one bit of difference to me.

My GP was very good and patient throughout my many visits. He then thought this was MS due to the combination of weird nervous system symptoms and my eyesight problems.

However, after a routine blood test he found I had an overactive thyroid and this threw him completely. This was causing classic symptoms of over activity, such as shaking, palpitations, sweating and the other symptoms. I had hardly noticed these problems however until they were pointed out to me. I found a book about thyroid disorders and read through the symptoms; most of my most irritating and upsetting problems were not listed. Although I was relieved to know that sweating was on the list, as I was beginning to think I would never wear a polo neck again! I was puzzled and really wanted more of an answer, in my mind I still had MS as the remaining symptoms were just like the list of MS symptoms I had read before.

I saw a specialist and once the thyroid was stable it became obvious I was still having the original set of symptoms and they were getting worse!

At times it felt as though I was the only person who knew this however I tried to explain it.

I found the most awful symptom was my worsening eyesight, it was so irritating. I could no longer read comfortably and the computer at work could reduce me to tears of frustration. Words would jump all over the page, letters all over the computer keyboard, I felt dizzy trying to keep up and concentrated so hard I would make my head ache.

At times it looked like there were raindrops all over the page obscuring parts of words by making them blurred, I would move my head trying to see around the 'drops'.

Very often I saw double and found it hard to coordinate my hand and eye movements, especially to type or do anything requiring me to look at close up. Seeing double is a very odd experience, which I still have at times even now. It seems to happen first thing in the morning, as if the eyes must get going.

My husband would bring me an early morning cuppa and I'd laugh and say, "I can see two of you!" He'd laugh back and say, "well there's only one cup of tea!" It was very weird at first however and I felt afraid until I knew what was causing the double vision.

I tried some magnifying glasses as an optician told me they would help me. I had a magazine in my car and rushed off with my glasses to read it, full of hope that I would be able to read comfortably again. I cried in the car park when I realised that my eyes were just the same as without the glasses.

My family tried to tell me I needed to get used to wearing glasses, but I knew they were a waste of time.

I often had visual disturbances lasting up to 30 minutes. These would appear as a flickering light in the corner of my vision, or zigzag shapes, or a cog shape. Even if I closed my eyes it was still visible.

These disturbances made me feel dizzy and I would feel the need to sit until it was over. At one time I was walking around the supermarket and the vision in the lower half of one eye just disappeared completely, all I could see from halfway down my line of vision was grey. This lasted a minute or so, then went away. The whole business was disconcerting to say the least, but also quite frightening.

My GP referred me to an eye specialist who found I had a problem with my eyes, not working together properly at close distances, he measured how bad it was. He said the eye problem was not typical of a thyroid problem and suggested an MRI scan to check for multiple sclerosis. He also gave me some eye exercises to do, which drove me crazy, but did seem to help a little.

Nothing abnormal was found by the MRI scan. I was desperate for an answer. I was pleased not to have MS but knew it was something. I knew the eye specialist felt I had a problem, but he couldn't just put his finger on what was causing it. He was kind but powerless to help me unless he knew the cause.

My memory became terrible and I would have trouble with forgetting the topic of conversation half way through talking. I did my best to cover this, but it felt like whatever this was it was taking me over; mind, body and soul. I would have to concentrate very hard all the time or lose the thread of what I was doing. I would drive a mile or two down the wrong road, then suddenly realise I was heading the wrong way.

I smiled on the outside, but I wept so much when I was alone, often when out in my car or out in the garden hidden by our willow tree. I even cried when the willow tree was pruned much to the amazement of my husband. The tree felt like a friend at that time, its hanging branches hid my shame at crying and sadness so well, and it briefly felt as though the world had ended when the branches were gone.

Later, I found it very apt that the tree regained its former glory at about the same time as I became better.

Feeling so ill was taking a serious toll now on my mental health as well. I needed to know why I felt ill and I needed others around me to know so that they would understand my anguish. It was a desperate and lonely time when I thought of little else but how ill and tired I felt. I really began to think I would die without anyone knowing why. Sometimes I wished I could just die, because I could see no light at the end of the tunnel and no end to my torment. Only thinking of my children really kept me determined to keep on.

My original consultant suggested I was depressed when I wept as I told him my symptoms, which perhaps I was, but only because I felt more ill than I had ever felt in my life and felt so alone. I refused anti-depressants and angrily told my own doctor that I was not depressed. He agreed and stayed firmly on my side, or at least if he had his doubts about my mental state he had the good grace not to mention them to me.

This was my lowest point. I was close to despair and often wept inconsolably but rarely when others could see. I didn't want my illness to be written off as depression and I could see if I gave in to my fears, in public too often, doubts would start settling into people's minds. Crying about my troubles had made one doctor say I was depressed, I was determined not to cry in front of another person if I could help it. That was my most terrible fear, I would be written off as a hypochondriac and depressive. I refused anti-depressants with fervour, as I knew they couldn't help me. Somehow, I needed to feel all my sadness and fear, not mask it. I knew it was a very real and not an imagined illness and I needed to keep everyone on my side. At times, the strain of this felt unbearable.

My GP kept me going more than he knows. His eyes were only showing concern and never, ever a moment of doubt, as I reeled off that week's problems!

I always felt he was my ally in this battle. I confessed to him that I often wept when alone and he said "and you say you aren't depressed?" He smiled as he said it because he knew what my reaction would be! I only had to say "don't you start" and he dropped the subject with a shake of his head and a smile.

I often kept a diary of my daily symptoms, as by now they were so weird I was trying to convince myself that it was real. One night my fingers on one hand went numb one by one and then gradually came back one by one as well, another time I couldn't undo some buttons on a child's shirt at the swimming pool as my coordination seemed all wrong.

My GP would read my diary and shake his head in puzzlement. I always felt that he wouldn't give up on me whatever happened, and I knew he would keep trying to find the answer however long it took.

I honestly think that his belief in me is the main factor that stopped me giving in and just dissolving into insanity. If he had once doubted my words in those awful times or been unkind I doubt my fragile mind could have taken the insult.

I have since heard such awful stories about the experiences of others with their doctors, that I realise how lucky I was to have an understanding one.

I felt everyone must have been getting fed up with this mystery illness. I longed for it to disappear and be all in my mind. I would have given almost anything for that to be true at that point.

I went to bed after tea; I sat in the bath for long spells trying to help the muscle pains. I couldn't carry heavy bags or hold a newspaper out to read it; my arms were like lead weights and ached continually. I couldn't read in any case, the words jumped all over the page. My arms ached when I drove the car, when shopping I had trouble deciding which was the worst option carrying my bags or walking back to the car to dump them, either way it was a trial. If something I needed was heavy I just couldn't buy it. Sometimes I felt rebellious and really forced myself to do heavy lifting, telling myself it was mind over matter. I would succeed but then feel so ill I needed to sit down and recover!

My leg or arm would suddenly feel numb and tingling, out of the blue, though I could still control the limb. My eyes thankfully were not affected by longer distance work like driving so I felt safe to do it still.

One day, I dropped a small bag of potatoes as a feeling like an electric shock ran down my arm. I had problems lifting saucepans when cooking and lifting a joint of meat out of the oven felt like weight training. Putting the empty milk bottles out, felt as though I was putting out full litre bottles of cola, everything felt so heavy.

My muscles in my thigh or calf would suddenly go into a spasm, it would take ages to get them moving again and it felt so frightening. Sometimes my fingers started twitching out of my control. I would look at them in horror and think, "what the hell is happening to me now?" My memory became so poor, it was like my mind was a thick fog that I had to wade through to recall things. I would do something and five minutes later had no recollection of it at all, however hard I tried to think.

I would be talking to someone and suddenly feel very distant, as though I was watching the scene from a long way away. It was as though my senses were on a dimmer switch and someone had turned it down a few notches. I could hide this, but it felt very strange and a little spooky!

I made silly mistakes at work, which made me feel I was losing control. I would spell things incorrectly or type the wrong word. I could stare at a word and not be able to tell if I had typed it correctly even though my spelling had always been a strong point.

Through all of this, OK I did look a little unwell, but with a little makeup I looked fine, and I kept smiling in public, so people assumed I *was* fine. I kept struggling on with my office job (luckily for me I worked for my husband, who sent me home lots of times when I couldn't cope and burst into tears.) Thank goodness that apart from one or two times when he lost patience with me, my husband faithfully stuck by me, (and all my troubles). I feel lesser men would have had enough of all the problems I had and left me. It never once seriously entered my head that my husband would ever desert me. I took my frustration out on him and my children with my nasty temper and tantrums, but it is a real credit to them that despite all of this they stuck by me and tried to help and understand. Illness and worry can literally change your personality. Other people outside my family expected me to carry on normally with my voluntary jobs and doing favours. I wasn't very good at refusing at that time either even though I felt at breaking point some days. I was used to being well and capable, I had always been the one to help others if I could and now I was having trouble doing the most mundane tasks for myself.

I felt guilty if I let people down and I remember being too ill to attend a village meeting. My telephone calls were met with disbelief when I said I was ill and the few people who I couldn't contact were annoyed at the meeting being cancelled without their knowledge, as they turned up to find the hall doors were locked.

I couldn't really see that this wasn't my fault and found myself apologising to people, as my head was spinning!

It's strange that being unwell is seen as a weakness and something to feel guilty about.

One desperate day when I felt I was in danger of falling into the well of despair and never surfacing again, I wrote in my diary in capitals I AM BRAVE AND STRONG AND ONE DAY EVERYONE WILL KNOW. They soon did, and I was the only one who had been expecting it.

Chapter 7

The Heart Attack, a miracle
and a name for my problems

One day in June 1999 I suddenly had a heart attack.

It was a busy morning and as I drove home I felt a pain in my chest, like indigestion. However, it very quickly got a lot worse and I knew I was having a heart attack. I felt strangely calm as I drove to the local surgery around the corner, parked the car and walked calmly in, saying good morning to an acquaintance as I went. As soon as I felt safe in the surgery I sunk to the floor in complete agony. My GP had another emergency chest pains patient with him whom he thought was a more likely candidate for a heart attack than me, so I had to wait until he had seen him.

After my ECG he realised, as unlikely as it seemed, I was the heart attack victim not his previous patient, a middle-aged man! My GP sent for the ambulance and at hospital I was treated with a clot buster and carefully watched for 24 hours in the cardiac unit. When I was asked whether I wanted the clot buster my head was spinning due to a Diamorphine injection for the pain.

The doctor told me that I needed the clot buster as I had almost certainly had a heart attack but once I had been given it I could bleed from anywhere in my body and they might not be able to stop it! For the first time I felt terrified, but I agreed.

I was in bed with this drug dripping into me and imagining that I would bleed to death at any moment but strangely again I became calm. The whole experience was surreal as though I was watching all this happening to someone else and they say I smiled the whole time. Perhaps it was the effect of the Diamorphine?

Once transferred to a ward I still received twice-daily Heparin injections and an aspirin each day.

On the second day a lady came around with library books. I explained that I couldn't see to read one, but the lady insisted I tried a large print book.

I gave in to get rid of her really.

To my amazement I could read, my eyes were totally clear! It was a miracle and I read constantly for the sheer joy of it. I felt ecstatic and puzzled but whatever the reason I didn't care.

When I'd recovered from the heart attack I was better than I'd been for a year or more. Most of my most unpleasant symptoms disappeared. There were ups and downs, but everyone understood now, and I had the perfect reason to say no. I took life easier, gave in to my illness, rested more and took long walks with my dog.

My only real problem was a pain which came and went in-between my shoulder blades. It felt at times like pressure or a tight band around me. I believed it was the after effects of the heart attack and tried to ignore it. I had the same pain in my leg muscles when I walked the dog and sometimes had to stop and rest until it passed.

Then one day in December 1999, whilst out shopping, I had a full-blown angina attack. I knew it wasn't a heart attack. Somehow, I knew if I could only sit down I'd be fine. The more I attempted to keep going, the worse I felt until I could no longer walk. However, I did drive home, which was silly, but I didn't realise that it was an angina attack and like most of us I didn't want to make a fuss.

I saw my doctor and then had an awful week on angina tablets and using an angina spray, but nothing made any difference. I finally gave in and saw my GP again. He sent me to the hospital where it was stated that it was unstable angina.

In hospital I was given an Isoket infusion, a drug that widened my arteries and relieved the pain. I had an angiogram, which showed I had completely clear arteries around my heart. Wide enough 'to drive double-decker buses down' they told me. It was suggested that I had Cardiac Syndrome X causing my arteries to tighten temporarily. While taking angina tablets to keep my blood vessels dilated I felt fine.

I was also tested for a clotting disorder; that was positive for the anticardiolipin antibodies. At this stage I wasn't told about this.

Six months later I was surprised to be asked to go for another blood test. This was also positive, and I saw the haematologist.

He told me very little about the illness. All he really wanted to know was whether I had any trouble with my pregnancies. When I said I had 4 children and no miscarriages he seemed to lose interest in me. He brushed aside the idea when I told him I'd had pre-eclampsia with my first and last pregnancies. He wasn't interested in any of my symptoms and just told me to take aspirin and watch out for thrombosis in my legs. However, I wanted to know everything. After all I'd been through I had to know so I asked him to write down the name.

He wrote LUPUS ANTICOAGULANT. I decided I would find out for myself on the internet as soon as I got home. For the first time I had an illness with a name and perhaps an answer to my strange symptoms and the heart attack. I felt both relieved and a little worried about what I would find out.

Chapter 8

The Internet

We hadn't had the Internet installed on our computer for very long, and I didn't have any experience of the World Wide Web. I just typed in 'Lupus Anticoagulant' as written on my scrap of paper. Incidentally to test positive for lupus anticoagulant, you don't have to have lupus and it promotes coagulation not anticoagulation. Aren't you glad you didn't come up with that name!

I came up with lots of sites about Antiphospholipid Syndrome also known as Hughes Syndrome. I soon realised that Lupus Anticoagulant was the name of a test for APS.

I found a wealth of information, chat rooms, a message forum, and Prof Graham Hughes on the St Thomas' Hospital lupus website. I also found Steve's page, which has the same title as the first chapter of this book, it was full of links to research and articles from all over the world about APS.

I was amazed that there were no books you could buy about this illness and nothing you could find in a library, but here on the internet I found a considerable amount of up to date information. For a week I read everything obsessively. Some of the information was quite frightening, other details made me feel vindicated. For the first time I realised none of this had been in my head; it was all very real and written in black and white.

After reading all the research and articles by Prof Hughes and his team at St Thomas' I became sure I should be taking Warfarin. I had tested positive, had the symptoms and had a major clotting incident. I began to see that without Warfarin I was taking an awful risk of another blood clot. My next thought was to ask how do I get the right treatment? And how would I persuade a doctor to go along with me?

I found the telephone number of a lady who set up the Hughes Syndrome Foundation, Hilary Clark. I rang the number and she was my turning point. It was her home number and there were children in the background. It was like chatting to a friend. She understood and identified with all that had happened to me. She also thought I should be taking Warfarin and suggested I should try to get a referral to see Prof Hughes.

I was excited now and begged my GP to get me there. It took him a few days and I was quietly going mad. I veered from complete faith that he would help me and being sure he would think me foolish and be annoyed.

Of course, he helped me, as I really knew he would, but hardly dared to take it for granted. He didn't think I could obtain treatment on the NHS but as I was insured he suggested we tried the private route.

When I saw my consultant (the one who had thought I was depressed) he also thought that seeing Prof Hughes was a great idea. It was a relief to feel I was doing the right thing and he was on my side. I forgave him for the depression incident and to his credit he never again mentioned depression to me.

Mind you, I was very careful that I never let my guard down and wept again!

Whilst I waited for my appointment with Prof Hughes I ended up back in hospital with unstable angina again. This time an enlightened young doctor had read all the latest about APS and couldn't understand why I wasn't taking Warfarin, as he said I tested positive for the antibodies and if a heart attack wasn't a major clotting incident what was? I could have hugged him. I was slowly discovering that doctors who understand APS are like gold dust, a rare breed to be treasured!

Of course, I agreed with him and he thought it was great I was going to see Prof Hughes. He hoped he had done what the man himself would do, by giving me Warfarin.

When I got home the angina became unstable again, so my doctor put my dose of artery widening drug up. This time, it worked.

Soon I would see Prof Hughes and I was taking Warfarin, I began to relax and feel safer. At last I was feeling positive about beating this illness, I knew what I was up against and it didn't stand a chance now. I couldn't help wondering what would have happened to me if I hadn't had the internet installed and if I hadn't been born with an overactive enquiring mind!

Chapter 9

Prof Graham Hughes - What a man!

After a long train journey to London and a taxi to the private clinic, I was finally at the door of Prof Graham Hughes' consulting room, with my husband.

As I entered I was surprised he wasn't taller. I'm not sure why but I imagined a big man and he wasn't. We shook hands and we all sat down. He told me to tell him everything from the start of it all.

He listened carefully, making notes as I talked, only interrupting to say, "how interesting," from time to time.

He was gentle and quietly spoken, his kindness was obvious.

Prof Hughes told me when I had finished that I had described the symptoms of Antiphospholipid Syndrome and the best thing for me was that I was taking Warfarin.

He said that if I had been taking it 10 years ago I would never have had a heart attack. He explained that without Warfarin the risk of another blood clot within the next 10 years was 50/50. There is a risk of bleeding with Warfarin but compared to the risk of disablement or death associated with a clot, it was not worth worrying about. He suggested I wore a Medic Alert necklace in case of any accident.

He advised me that my Warfarin treatment should be life-long whatever the antibodies did, as the benefits far outweighed the risks. He said that if I did this I would be home and dry. These words were so uplifting, and I often tell myself when life seems difficult that I'm 'home and dry', it never fails to cheer me up!

After he had examined me he told us of his research with Multiple Sclerosis patients. He and his team had discovered a percentage of MS sufferers had the APS antibodies. When these people were treated with Warfarin their symptoms improved or went completely. What a breakthrough and how wonderful for those lucky people! Of course, having APS is no fun, but it is an infinitely better prospect than multiple sclerosis, which has no known cure and is a progressively debilitating condition in many cases.

He went on to tell us of a lady who had gone blind in one eye and was losing the sight in her second eye. She was referred to him when they discovered she had the APS antibodies and once she was given Warfarin therapy her eyesight was fully restored. This explained my miracle after my heart attack, my blood was thinned, therefore my eyesight improved.

Depression is another popular diagnosis to describe APS patients. We have such strange and varied symptoms it is understandable that some doctors assume it is all in the mind. Prof Hughes told me of a patient whose memory had got so bad she forgot to collect her children from school. The nurse who took my blood test afterwards told me of a lady doctor with this illness who was sectioned under the Mental Health Act and put into a psychiatric hospital for a time before she was eventually tested for APS.

Prof Hughes saw me twice a year. I now have been diagnosed as suffering from Hughes Syndrome, Sjogren's, Autoimmune Thyroid Disease, type 2 diabetes and Cardiac Syndrome X, so my life is not really as it was before. I work part time and get along fine really within the constraints of my illness.

As for Prof Hughes, I can honestly say he is one of the kindest, least pompous and most dedicated doctors I have ever met. When we left his consulting room, I just turned to my husband and said, "wasn't he lovely?" My husband could only agree.

As time has gone by, my admiration for this man has increased.

I have read about the endless work he has done in the field of Lupus and Hughes Syndrome research.

My APS friends in America, whom I meet in the various forums and groups are envious that I see 'the man' himself! However, Prof Hughes has no idea of how much he is worshipped from afar, a friend told him she felt as though she'd had an audience with God! She told me that Prof Hughes just looked a little puzzled. He would be so surprised that so many people all over the world are in awe of him.

He is so patient and makes time for everyone that he can. His enthusiasm for helping his patients and researching APS is infectious. He has helped me with this book and with other APS projects with which I have been involved. He has readily agreed to being interviewed by the lowliest of news reporters to get publicity for the illness at both a local and national level, (at international level as well I guess!) and charms them all.

A couple of times I have telephoned his secretary and ended up chatting to Prof Hughes himself. I understand this was a common occurrence, he was more accessible than my local doctors! Many of the people who worked for or with him were patients; I can understand why anyone would want to work alongside him.

I have never heard anyone who sees him regularly speak ill of him; he always seems to be courteous and kind. I will never understand how he fits everything in.

Everyone who knows this man agrees he is an inspiration.

After he retired he still saw private patients for a few years. He still works hard to spread awareness of the condition even now that he is in his late 70s and retired.

What a hero!

Chapter 10

Things that are hard to talk about

There are some aspects of Hughes Syndrome which are hard to talk about, as they are so feared. A book about the illness would not be complete without mentioning these, however hard we find it to discuss things that frighten us. It is only fair to those friends I have made through the internet who have suffered so badly that we find the courage to face the most worrying aspects of Hughes Syndrome.

Catastrophic Antiphospholipid Syndrome

This is a major medical emergency. For some reason the APS can crank up a gear or two very suddenly. When this problem occurs blood clots form at random, affecting limbs, internal organs, in fact just about any part of the body. This is very much more serious than a single clot as there can be many clots all at once stopping the blood flow to just about anywhere.

Naturally a person with catastrophic APS very quickly becomes seriously ill and needs intensive care.

Thankfully this is a very rare complication of APS.

It is in fact so rare that there are no definite figures for survival but with specialist treatment it is possible to come through.

The Causes?

The causes of this rare complication are not really known yet, but it is often after anticoagulation treatment has gone wrong in some way. This can happen after a traumatic event; a car crash or operation when Warfarin is discontinued temporarily because of the risk of bleeding.

Sometimes it seems to occur when triggered by an infection. It can also happen when anticoagulation is stopped by a well-meaning doctor, often just to see what happens!

What can we do to protect ourselves?

This may be very rare, but we need to be as safe as we can be from it.

My suggestions are:

- To wear a Medic Alert bracelet always, with details of your APS doctor and as much detail on the bracelet as can be fitted on the disc.

- Secondly, never allow any doctor to stop the anticoagulation without your APS specialist agreeing to it. (It is highly unlikely that a knowledgeable doctor would stop anticoagulation at all anyway). I was told once when in hospital to miss a dose of Warfarin as my INR was 4. I refused and explained that 4 was fine for me. The doctor argued with me and I threatened to discharge myself as her advice would make me more ill or possibly kill me. She gave in eventually, it wasn't fun but sticking up for what you know is correct is the only way.

- Thirdly, only have surgery if it is to save your life or you feel your life is not worth living without an operation. Cosmetic reasons are not worth it, and I would rather put up with lots of medical problems than have surgery unnecessarily. If surgery is your only option, then discuss it carefully with your doctor and surgeon. Lots of APS patients have surgery, and there are no problems as a result. With careful anticoagulation management you should be fine.

- Lastly be very careful about which medications you take as well as Warfarin. Always tell those treating you that you take Warfarin. Ladies should be very aware that hormone treatment, of any kind, is really to be avoided at all costs. Herbal medicines and natural remedies can affect your INR also, so never take anything without checking first with your doctor.

Treatment

Because this aspect of Hughes Syndrome is so rare treatment is not really a definite science.

Anticoagulation seems to be the most important treatment. Some doctors also try plasma exchange to clean the antibodies from the blood; this however has yet to be proved as an effective treatment. New research comes up with new treatments however so perhaps soon more will be understood.

Survivors of Catastrophic APS

I will mention no names in this section as the people mentioned are understandably sensitive about their problems.

I know of three survivors of this problem. I'm positive that there are many more than the ones I know about. One sufferer had severe clotting in his heart, brain and other organs. He is left with severe disabilities, which he deals with cheerfully most of the time. He is unable to work but devotes a lot of time to helping others with APS through the internet and lives as full a life as possible.

The other two were both female, one has had her leg amputated because of an inexperienced doctor's treatment and another had to have a mastectomy.

The tissue starved of oxygen by clots died and removal of the affected areas was their only choice.

Both young (in their 30s) these ladies cope as well as they can. Understandably they are not always cheerful, but they manage and do all they can to help and advise others with APS.

These people are now coping by taking anticoagulation treatment. One still has ongoing problems that I know of caused mainly by the incorrect treatment she initially received.

She is so brave, and I really hope that her experience of how terrifyingly serious this illness can be will stand as a warning to us all to look after ourselves and speak out.

Perhaps if they had all been anticoagulated before and all through their ordeals they could have been saved their permanent reminder of how ill they have been.

For the sake of those who survive the worst that APS can throw at us, and the sake of those unknown who have died, I hope that this chapter has made the reader think carefully about protecting themselves.

Never put up with symptoms such as blue toes or leg ulcers. (OK, I know that might sound strange, but some have ignored such obvious signs, so that's why I said it!) Always report strange occurrences however petty it may seem when you see your doctor.

Most importantly never go along with something you believe to be wrong just to keep the peace or not to cause trouble to others.

It is your life so speak out however difficult or awkward it may be, however much you may feel in awe of doctors, and be quite prepared and determined to always be in control of what is done to your body. I have threatened to discharge myself from hospital before. Speak up, be determined to be heard.

Most of us will be fine on Warfarin and never develop any of this so perhaps it is best not to dwell on it. If everything you can do to protect yourself is done, then getting on with life is the best option.

Some things we cannot control so we must do the best we can and then forget it, to keep our sanity!

Chapter 11

How to deal with doctors

This is not a section about doctor bashing. When your illness is not well known or understood, you come to realise there are three types of doctors.

The first is the one that has never heard of your illness or has limited knowledge but will listen to you and read the information you have carefully printed from the internet. Although they are not knowledgeable about your unusual illness, they are willing to learn along with you and are open to your suggestions. They will usually refer you to a specialist.

The second is the doctor who professes to know all about these blood-clotting illnesses but when you listen to what he tells you, your heart sinks. They may be hopelessly out of date, or worse. This type of doctor is very hard to convince of the need for a referral. Often, they will dismiss your carefully printed information as nonsense from the internet.

Some go as far as to say most of this is all in your head and perhaps suggest that you should read less about your illness when in fact they really should read more! If this type of doctor refuses to listen (you must have a try at talking to him/her) my suggestion is to keep your cool but refuse to ever see them again. Ask for another referral and if you feel strongly enough order a copy of Prof Hughes book and send it to the original doctor with the polite suggestion that they should read it! If you can afford the cost of the book it is a worthy investment as they will perhaps take their next APS patient more seriously.

In fact, Prof Hughes' books are a good buy, if only to convince doctors of the seriousness of this illness, they won't take my book seriously overall as I am a mere patient sadly! Prof Hughes' vast knowledge of the ways in which this illness can affect his patients means that anything he writes about APS is interesting to read. His charity website www.ghic.world is also very helpful. It is well worth a look and it covers Lupus and Hughes Syndrome.

The last type of doctor is that wonderful person who has read all the current thinking about Hughes Syndrome, understands how important it is that you are treated and never ever tells you that it is "in your mind"! This is a doctor that all people with Hughes Syndrome should see but sadly sometimes it can be a battle to get there.

I will imagine that you are new to the illness and have been diagnosed. You have read all about Hughes Syndrome on the internet and feel afraid because you are not taking any anticoagulants. The main thing is not to panic. A calm patient is more likely to be listened to than a worked up, agitated one.

The first thing is to get your GP on side. The best way is to print a few articles from good sources on the internet (from reliable and reputable sources). Write a short note to your GP asking them to read these articles prior to your appointment, as you feel you need to see a specialist.

This way when you tell your GP that you have Hughes Syndrome or Antiphospholipid Syndrome they will not be thrown into a panic wondering what that is, and you will not make them feel foolish.

Making a doctor feel foolish is not the best way to get the help you desperately need.

When you see them calmly say that you feel that having read current research you are at risk from another blood clot without anticoagulation. Then ask if they would mind considering the possibility of a referral, if you can find a good specialist yourself, get the hospital address and their name and have them ready.

If your doctor is unhelpful try not to blow your top. Just calmly say that you would like to change your GP unless they are willing to investigate the illness further or refer you to someone who knows more. Explain that it is your life that you are discussing, and you are unwilling to risk disability or death for the want of a referral. I read recently about a person who says to any doctor who refuses them a referral "Can you please put in my notes that you refused to help me."

If this doesn't move them you will have to try again with a new GP, but in these days, it is a brave or foolish doctor who dismisses you out of hand.

Once you have been taken seriously and are taking Warfarin (if that is what is needed in your case) the next problems may arise at the anticoagulation clinic.

It can be a problem to convince doctors that your INR needs to be as high as 3 or even 3.5 or even higher. They fear that you will bleed incessantly. You need to be very firm and insistent. If they refuse to up your dose to achieve a high enough INR tell your specialist immediately that you are having problems. A letter from them will soon sort out any fears that the clinic doctors may have.

Always take responsibility for your INR, you should always know your last test result. You should also have a card with all your recent results listed. These days you may have an e mail with your results but always have the result of your last test with you.

Never rely on a doctor or other health worker to tell you if there's a problem, ask for the actual INR result yourself every time you are tested. If you think your dose should go up then say so, whether the doctor in charge likes it or not. I had one doctor who ended up asking me what I thought about my dose every time I went! I didn't mind at all and we got on very well! He would smile and raise his eyebrows every time he saw me. I was very sorry when he left the clinic, I wonder if the feeling was mutual?

If you feel there is too long between your blood tests then say so, you don't have to do as you are told, you can have an opinion.

It is important to remain calm, know your stuff and be as pleasant as you can about it. Doctors are under lots of stress and an awkward patient who shouts at them is not really someone they feel like being reasonable with. They are more likely to think you are a neurotic hypochondriac, sadly being female still seems to make this more likely. I know that sticking your neck out and speaking up can be difficult but there is no need to lose your temper or be unpleasant. If you are polite and insistent it is more effective. A smiling patient, who calmly says "would you mind if I gave you my opinion?" is more likely to be listened to by any reasonable worthwhile doctor.

This is all very hard when you feel so ill but unfortunately until Hughes Syndrome is better understood and known it is the only way. All we really want is to feel that the doctors are in charge and know what is best but unfortunately sometimes you must take charge of your own life, whether you feel up to it or not.

It is important to remember that doctors cannot be expected to know everything. It is up to all of us to educate those who need it, for the sake of their next Hughes Syndrome patient.

Chapter 12

Heredity

Hughes Syndrome is only vaguely hereditary, in a similar way to diabetes. In some families there seems to be a strong link with different generations having blood-clotting problems but in others there doesn't seem to be anyone else. Why this is, is yet unknown. Sometimes Hughes Syndrome can cluster in a family, sometimes only show up in far-removed relatives.

What could be hereditary is the tendency to develop an autoimmune illness of some sort but even so there is little evidence to support what remains little more than guesswork. I suspect my maternal grandmother had Hughes Syndrome as she had heart attacks in her 50s and was put on Warfarin. My son has Psoriasis which is autoimmune. It seems more of a family tendency rather than being directly passed on.

There is current research into how heredity may be involved. Hopefully it will help us to understand how the illness works.

The reason most of us want to know about this is that we have children and we are anxious to know that we have not passed on this illness to them.

So, a question is raised. Whether to get your children tested or not?

My view is that if your child is showing symptoms that you recognise, such as migraines or vision problems then get them tested. It is better to know than sit around worrying needlessly or worse sit around waiting for a blood clot. Knowing must be better than burying your head in the sand.

If you have a daughter who is considering taking the contraceptive pill it is better to know and be safe than spend a lifetime regretting a decision to hope for the best.

If your child needs an operation and you are concerned that they are showing signs of Hughes Syndrome, then don't panic about blood clots just ask for the test before the operation. After all you must give your permission for the operation to take place, so speak out.

It is likely that the tests will be negative and then you can forget about your worries. Even if it is a positive result you will know what to do and which doctor to see. It is not the end of the world, just great that it is picked up in plenty of time and can be monitored.

You know the signs now, so you will notice any member of future generations who seem to have familiar symptoms and you will be the wise old relative with all the answers. I hope that by the time my grandchildren grow up no one will die from this illness. So much has been discovered since I was first diagnosed I feel sure that Hughes Syndrome in the future will be managed much as diabetes is now.

Chapter 13

How to cope with Hughes Syndrome

I will try to tell you my ways of coping, but as we are all different perhaps they won't help in your case. I can only do my best.

It always helps me to remember there are people all over the world struggling with this syndrome, just as I do. The internet is useful in this respect as you can speak in groups to others with similar problems to your own and so learn how they cope. Facebook has some great groups.

There is such a variation in how this illness affects people's lives. Some are completely unable to do many day-to-day tasks, others can carry on as normal once treated, and it seems that most fall somewhere between those two extremes with awful days and ok days and occasional fit days.

There is always someone with more to cope with than you. This is very true with APS.

I have spoken to Patrick on the internet since he was 21. He has been in a wheelchair since he had a stroke at 16.

I had previously thought I was a young sufferer, but he put it into perspective for me. He is always cheerful. He works and rarely wallows in self-pity.

We have lots of laughs at completely unrelated subjects and I think if he can cope so cheerfully, so can I. His catchphrase is 'never give up'.

He is now married with children and getting on with life as cheerfully as ever.

I also speak to Lynette, who had a 6-year-old daughter with APS who had a stroke. She stayed positive and almost never dwelt on how sad the situation was. Her daughter has now grown up and deals with her illness as we all do. She has made Lynette very proud.

This is the great thing about adversity. If we don't let it beat us it makes us stronger.

I must admit though that when I'm feeling very ill I don't care about anyone else's problems, so that theory doesn't always stand up to scrutiny.

Understanding family and friends are needed more than anything else. If yours don't understand, give them this book to read, so they know what you deal with. You must remember however that it is impossible for them to know how you feel. They have never felt that tired or ill, except when they have had the flu, in most cases. How can they understand that you live with this weariness continually or how awful that can be without being there themselves? Stop fighting the thoughtlessness of others and excuse them, as always standing on a soapbox or moaning will just exhaust you and is pointless. Only another person with a long-term illness can understand feeling so tired that feeding the dog and hanging a shirt out to dry can leave you feeling as though you just ran a marathon.

At times it all gets too much to bear. A bad day, a lot of pain, or a thoughtless comment can tip the scales the wrong way sometimes. Stress is the number one thing to try to avoid as much as possible. I know it's difficult and there will always be stress but don't go looking for it. If someone constantly gives you stress, consider whether you need them in your life. Don't get drawn into other's problems. If you put your own feelings first it isn't a sin, it's necessary to stay well and not be a nuisance to your nearest and dearest.

Don't let worries build up. Tell someone and try to solve the problem. Constant fears, worry and resentments can lead to stress and stress leads to more illness. Stress is not a psychological thing. It is physical. Hormones are released when you are stressed and prolonged exposure to this can cause physical illness. Cut anyone who causes you to be constantly on edge out of your life. I had to cut my own mother out of mine many years ago and though it is sad that I had to, it has been the best thing ever for my health.

Give in to tiredness, a well-timed snooze can change the whole outlook of the day. One girl described the tiredness by saying that your energy is a jar of coins, on a good day they last you all day as you spread out your spending. On a bad day they are all gone by lunch and you have no alternative but to give in and rest. Sometimes you can borrow some coins from tomorrow, but you always end up having to pay them back with an easy day! An example of this is when I danced till late at a party and ended up sleeping most of the next day. Still it was worth it! I still do this knowing that I will pay for it as I need to live my life and not stop doing everything I enjoy.

If work is becoming impractical you may be forced to give up or work part time. As hard as that makes your life remember that at least you can be of use looking after the house or the children. If you work until you are ill, you will help no one. Don't let that happen, give in as gracefully as you can. A partner who does a little gardening and sorts out household matters at their own pace, beats one who is always in hospital!

Accept all offers of help even if you think you don't need it, or you think people are fussing. You may be grateful for that saved energy later in the day. Be gracious and grateful, people like to help, so let them.

Exercise and eat sensibly. Lose weight if you can and you need to. I keep battling on with that one!

No crash dieting with the Warfarin though.

Smoking is bad, and I won't preach but trust me when I say it is the worst thing you can do.

Have one or two drinks but don't get drunk! It plays havoc with Warfarin and if you already feel as though you have a hangover imagine the next day!

On a bad day, be kind to yourself and leave things.

On a good day, make the most of it and do whatever you like the most!

Don't allow yourself to be dumped on by well-meaning folk who think you have lots of spare time.

There are lots of fit people who can do the committee things and charity collections. Do only what you want to do and feel up to doing.

When you look well, those around you may forget you are struggling. Remind them in a cheerful way that you are feeling ill or tired. It is so easy to get forgotten when you have rosy cheeks and look fitter than most. We don't wish to look ill, but it would help sometimes when we feel ill!

Sometimes the most hurtful comment can simply be when someone says, "But you look so well". It is usually well meant but when you feel very ill and tired it can seem like a total lack of understanding of what you are going through. My usual response is, "Yes and that is half of my problem, if I looked ill it would be easy for you to understand." Although if I can't be bothered to get on my soapbox, I just smile and let it go.

You need to remember that you still have a life to live even with long-term illness. Do as much as you are able to. Never worry what others may think if you are out dancing on a good night, you don't have to live as an ill person, just because you feel ill one day, it doesn't mean that you will not feel fine the next.

Book that holiday and plan evenings out. Never worry about not feeling well enough. If you are ill on the day, then you can cancel but the chances are you'll be fine and have the time of your life. Try not to think of yourself as an ill person but one with a disability, which restricts you now and then. If people get too wrapped up in the role of an ill person, it will make them miserable and left out. Try to go for it!

Don't panic about the scarier parts of APS. Once I read a very black report on the internet about a poor long-term prognosis for those with APS. It said that most patients with APS had major organ damage and were long-term disabled due to damage before anticoagulation and in general the long-term prognosis was poor.

I thought, "Oh no, I'm going to be disabled," and felt so worried for a little while. Then I thought, "Just a minute, I have major organ damage from my heart attack and I am now considered to be long-term disabled because of my angina". I also realised that my poor memory could count as a disability and that I was unable to work full time. A wave of relief came over me when I realised that I was already disabled! I was also fine and living a very happy life so what was I so afraid of? On paper things look much more frightening than when faced in reality.

Now I'm used to it, as strange as it sounds I don't want to go back to being the person I used to be before I was ill. At first that was all I longed for, to return to my old self. This experience has changed me, made me more tolerant and patient. I no longer worry about the finer details of life but go with the flow so much more. When someone sounds their car horn at me I smile and think how sad to spend your life getting angry about unimportant things. Having a disability can reveal your true self, and you may find there are different sides to your personality you had never had the time to notice before. There is time to see the flowers now whereas before I would have only seen the weeding!

Don't put off doing anything. Perhaps waiting until the kids are older or until there is more money or until there is more time. If you really want to do something then go for it, book that holiday, go to see your favourite band, live life. Life is only here and now, even more so for us than most others, so live every day that you can, doing what you really want to do, if possible.

I hope this book has helped. If it helps just one person I will know this illness was for a reason and not just to irritate me. After all I always loved to write but never did until now. At least this illness inspired me to do something about that. This book is not intended to be a collection of experiences, but three important people should be recognised, and one way is to let them tell their stories.

Hilary Clark is founder of the Hughes Syndrome Foundation. Hilary was the person who saved my life by telling me I needed to see Prof Hughes. She must have done the same for so many others whilst she ran the foundation from her home.

Over the years the need for help grew and eventually the charity was formed, based at St Thomas' Hospital. The following is her story.

She says; "I was six months pregnant with my first child when I had my first blood clot in my leg. Fortunately, I gave birth to a healthy baby boy on the 8th of September 1986.

I had a history of migraine attacks, which continued through pregnancy and beyond. I also developed varicose veins, circulation problems, and bouts of chronic tiredness, with steadily worsening discolouration on my feet.

In 1991 developed a DVT in my right leg and spent a week in hospital on an intravenous Heparin drip. On discharge I was prescribed Warfarin for three months and told that the probable cause of the clot had been the contraceptive pill I had been taking.

Between 1989 and 1994 I suffered from bouts of phlebitis, swollen ankles, migraine attacks, chronic tiredness and pain in my legs. In 1994 whilst nine weeks pregnant with my second child, I developed a blood clot, again in my right leg. Given my history, my GP started me on a course of Heparin injections to thin my blood. I was also tested for Lupus and antiphospholipid antibodies. Whilst the test for Lupus was negative I had tested positive for APS (Hughes Syndrome). I was then referred to a haematologist at my local hospital, who prescribed 2,500 units of Heparin per day and continued to monitor my blood.

During my 30-week antenatal appointment my doctor was unable to find my baby's heartbeat. I was driven to the hospital where a scan confirmed that my baby had died. I gave birth to Liam two days later 28th of January 1995.

During the two weeks that followed, while we waited for our baby's body to be returned after post-mortem, I developed another DVT. After Liam's funeral, I was admitted to hospital, where I was again given heparin through a drip. We later learned that Liam had died due to blood clots that had formed in my placenta, which had starved him of food and oxygen.

Throughout this time my GP was wonderful. She treated my depression, helped me receive counselling and persuaded me to attend Prof Hughes' clinic at St Thomas' Hospital; after reading an article on his work. In October 1995 I met with Prof Hughes and became one of his patients.

After losing Liam, I had been consumed with guilt and confusion. I felt so isolated. I needed information about my condition, to understand what had caused my body to kill my baby. I needed to know how to manage this syndrome; I needed to feel in control. I was desperate to talk to someone who understood; someone who had been through the dark tunnel that I had and who could walk me through to the other side. There was no one. I decided to start a support line from my home, to save others from the despair that I had felt. With the help of my health visitor, Ronnie Bray, on the 28th of January 1996, a year to the day since Liam had been born; the Hughes Syndrome Foundation was started.

In preparation for another pregnancy I attended Prof Hughes and Dr Khamashta's clinic in the autumn of 1996. I was prescribed 5,000 units of heparin, which I injected twice a day. I was also given baby aspirin to take daily.

In the January of 1997 I became pregnant and this time my pregnancy was closely monitored via my GP and local hospital, overseen by St Thomas'. I attended the clinic at St Thomas' every three months for blood tests, check-ups, Doppler flow scans, and scans to check my baby's progress. Although success was not guaranteed, I always came away from the clinic with a very real sense of optimism. On the 26th September 1997 I gave birth to my daughter Lara. She was born two weeks early by caesarean section, healthy and perfect.

I have been migraine and DVT free since 1995.

I will have to take Warfarin for the rest of my life and my blood is regularly monitored. I control my muscle pain with a combination of codeine and paracetamol and manage my energy levels the best I can. I still suffer bouts of extreme tiredness and brain fog. Sometimes when I am struggling to find a word my brain substitutes it with another word by association. Those who know me best are used to this and laugh with me. Sometimes my mind will freeze, like a computer screen, and I will momentarily forget what I am talking about. I know that overall, people with this condition suffer far more than I have, and I count my blessings. I hope in time with more access to help and information, that diagnoses will be made earlier and the correct treatment given sooner, which will lessen the suffering.

I like to think Liam's death was for a reason. If it hadn't been for my experiences through losing him, I wouldn't have been able to help as many people in the way that I have. I feel proud to be a part of the growing awareness of this condition and privileged to have been able to help.

Being asked to contribute to this book reminded me that I am not alone, and that it isn't in my head, as I am sure we all tend to find ourselves thinking from time to time. I am sure that this book will help others to better understand this condition, whilst also helping those of us who live with it."

Mark Waxman Founder of the Delphi APS Forum says: "In 1993, I was diagnosed with Hughes. It has caused me several heart attacks, DVT's and a double pulmonary embolism. To learn more about my disorder I created a website and an online forum to help myself and others to learn more and, in that process, have been in contact with hundreds of patients, relatives and their friends with questions about Hughes. Of all the things we had in common, one stood out, we wanted a guide, a book on what our disorder was, what it meant. We weren't happy with being a footnote in a medical reference guide. We wanted something written in terms we could understand and relate to, something we could hold in our hands, something we could share with others. With this book, Kay has accomplished that goal. She has written clearly and concisely from a patient's point of view, doing the research necessary. Kay has done a wonderful job in explaining what it means to live with Hughes. If you have Hughes, or know someone who does, this book is an invaluable guide." My dear friend Mark sadly died in 2015 from APS.

Lynette Stewart (joint founder of the internet e group APLSUK) has a particularly moving story; "At the beginning of 1999 my daughter, who was four and a half years old at the time, complained of sore ears, so I took her to the doctors who checked her ears out and said that they were both a bit red and gave me some antibiotics for her.

That was the first of four visits to the doctors in a week, as my daughter seemed to be getting worse.

My fourth visit to the doctor was an emergency because my daughter woke up on a Monday morning with the left-hand side of her face completely swollen and foul-smelling pus coming out of her left ear.

We were sent to the ENT clinic at our local hospital and my daughter was admitted to hospital the same day. On the Wednesday my daughter had surgery to remove the mastoid from behind her left ear, because she had severe Otitis Media (middle ear infection). Apparently, it is very rare to perform this type of surgery on a child so young, so my daughter was put in the ICU (Intensive Care Unit) overnight for observation.

Thursday was the beginning of a journey, which changed my life forever. I can't remember what time it was on the Thursday morning, but the nurse who was monitoring my daughter suddenly became very concerned, when my daughter started shaking several times down the right-hand side of her body.

She disappeared and then several different doctors appeared back with the nurse, one of the doctors tested my daughter's reflexes in her arms, legs, feet and hands, there was no response.

I was taken to another room, and my husband was telephoned. When he arrived, doctors said they didn't know what was wrong with our daughter and the PICU (Paediatric Intensive Care Unit) from another hospital was coming to retrieve her.

My daughter was finally taken to the PICU where she had a lumbar puncture and other tests, all which seemed ok. She was on a ventilator to help her to breathe, was tube fed and was covered in other tubes providing medication.

A nurse took photographs of my daughter as it would be a good idea for my three sons to see what their sister looked like before they visited. Jonathan, a young trainee doctor, noticed that it looked as though her swollen face had dropped a little.

Jonathan was puzzled so there were more tests, which showed she had thrombosis of the jugular vein, and thrombosis of the cavernous sinus.

Then followed even more tests to find out why she had thrombosis. An MRI scan showed that she had a partial infarction of the brain.

I was told that day by a doctor to prepare myself for my daughter to die and if by some miracle she did live she would be a vegetable for the rest of her life.

I broke down and cried my eyes out and then managed to phone my husband (who was decorating the bungalow we had just bought), I told him what the doctor had said to me and heard him scream no at the top of his voice. My husband assured me he would come to the hospital straight away, but he needed to see our three sons first to let them know he was coming to the hospital.

My father, who lives in Cambridge, drove through the night to arrive at the hospital around 2am.

We spent all night sitting with our daughter, thinking are we going to lose her. Wondering what will she be like if she does survive?

The tests came back to show that my daughter had Anticardiolipin antibodies in her blood stream and she was given aspirin as the neurologist thought she was too young for Warfarin as it could make her bleed more easily.

Over a week later she came off the ventilator. It had been tried earlier but each time she suffered strokes. This time however she was breathing unaided. During this period the physiotherapists applied casts to her legs and feet. Her feet were extended and the casts, which were changed every few days, were intended to bring her feet back to a normal position.

Away from the ventilator she began to start a mouthing motion (biting inside her mouth and lips).

One day as I went to cuddle her the nurse said she had bitten inside her mouth again. As I got a tissue to wipe away the blood I realised it wasn't just blood, part of her tongue was hanging from the corner of her mouth. I was in a state of shock and so was the nurse, it affected the both of us, the nurse and me, so much that we both went home for the rest of the day.

Then dentists made mouth guards for her upper and lower teeth (very similar to the ones rugby players wear) and it was suggested that all her teeth would be removed if she continued the mouthing motion.

She was later moved from the PICU to another ward. It was a couple of days after this a nurse noticed her skin was bright red and when we lifted her arms clumps of skin were peeling off (she looked as though she had been badly sunburnt). The dermatology department found she was allergic to one of her medicines, which was stopped immediately, and the allergic reaction slowly disappeared.

During this time, she was spitting her mouth guards out and pulling the nasal tube that was feeding her, making her nostrils bleed.

It was decided to remove the mouth guards, and a doctor wanted to insert a tube direct into her stomach to feed her. The dietician had other ideas and said we should try my daughter on foods like yoghurt and try to work our way up slowly.

One day a nurse was talking to my daughter who repeated the words, "good girl". She then repeated the phrase. I was overjoyed as she had been in hospital for eight weeks by this time, and this was the first sign of progress.

We took it one step at a time, and I showed her photos of her dad and brothers asking her who they all were, and she named every one of them.

I was thankful that her mind was intact, and she knew who we all were. We fell into a daily routine.

Often at night she would wake up screaming, and I would sit with her until she calmed down and finally went back to sleep.

She was getting stronger by the day, moving from yoghurts to very mashed up food. Peas didn't seem to mash very well and one stuck in her throat one day making her sick (she still doesn't like peas to this day).

She started school within the hospital, and that came as a relief, as she began to join in and use the computer.

One day I took her in a wheelchair just so she could get some fresh air and walking round the local town, I found how hard it is to get into some shops with a wheelchair, it was a nightmare and after an hour we returned to the hospital.

We then had a wonderful weekend at home. The weather was glorious, and we went to the school fair at my youngest son's school. We saw people we hadn't seen for months, my daughter saw her friends from play school, she had the biggest smile on her face that I have ever seen.

Weeks later she was transferred to our local hospital for a week where we found the staff had been telephoning every day for news of her progress. Somehow my daughter had proved the doctor who said she would die or if by some miracle she did live she would be a vegetable for the rest of her life wrong.

She was given a walker to help her walk and special shoes and she graduated from the leg casts to a leg splint on her right leg.

After another week in hospital she came home, we had spent a total of 18 or 19 weeks in hospital altogether.

Every week we were back at the hospital for appointments with the physiotherapist, the occupational therapist, speech therapist, hearing specialist, eye specialist, paediatrician and neurologist. Then came visits from the special needs medical teachers to see which school she would attend. Eventually they decided she could go to the same school as my youngest son.

In September she started school in a wheelchair and was wearing nappies (because she had lost control of her bladder and bowels).

After the first full day it was decided she should attend for just part of the day and I would go to school with her until the school could employ a full-time assistant to be with her.

By November she was potty trained and didn't use her walker any longer. Her walking back to school after half term was a surprise to everyone.

She was often frustrated, so much so that I could end up with black, blue and purple bruises all over my left arm.

At one appointment with the paediatrician and neurologist I asked what Anticardiolipin antibodies were. They did not answer and at each subsequent visit I kept asking the same questions without ever receiving a sensible reply. This made me angry and I decided to do some research on the internet and found the APS Forum at Delphi run by Mark Waxman and another online group for people who have Auto Immune Diseases.

I read about Antiphospholipid Syndrome and talked to people via the internet who suffered with APS. It was a godsend as finally I was talking to people who understood what I was talking about and knew what my daughter had been through.

With my friend Patrick I started APLSUK (which is an international internet support group), on January 14th, 2001. Although we are both members of the Delphi Forum, we felt that there was the need and the room for another support group, where we could share ideas, information, offer help and support to people who suffer with APS, and their families and friends.

Patrick and I spent countless hours talking to each other via the Internet. He is the same age as my oldest son and to my surprise and astonishment totally understood everything that I was talking about, which was wonderful.

Today we have over 200 members in our family (as I like to think we are an APS family) in 15 different countries. We have nurses, priests, a paramedic, a scientist, housewives and business people in our family.

Most members suffer with APS, and some are carers of husbands, wives and children who suffer with APS. There was great joy when one of our members in Australia gave birth to a baby boy a few months ago after suffering a string of heart-breaking miscarriages.

We now also have a sister group; started by a family member of APLSUK for those ladies in our family who have suffered miscarriages due to APS.

Now you may be asking how my daughter is today. She is a fighter, who is now 8 years old and in the first year of the juniors at school and she is a Brownie. She does have problems; motor co-ordination, visual and hearing impairment, short-term memory loss and the partial infarction of the brain has caused emotional and behavioural problems. She can ride a bike but needs stabilisers and cannot use a skipping rope.

Despite her problems she lives her life like a normal child of eight years old and I am very proud of everything she has achieved since she was taken ill when she was four and a half years old. Everyone, who has APS or has a relative with APS, has walked down a long road and through the darkness alone in a search for knowledge about APS.

As corny as you may think it is, we all do have "Faith of the Heart" a Rod Stewart song that sums up my feelings about this illness and how we have been affected by it."

Happily, Lynette's daughter is grown up, in her 20s and managing well in 2018. The groups she ran are now replaced with Facebook groups.

As a footnote to this chapter I would like to say that Mark Waxman was a force for good for everyone with APS. I felt his INR was kept too low to protect him but didn't realise this until it was too late. He had extensive damage to his heart caused by his many heart attacks and his body could take no more. He fought so bravely, and I miss him and his wise words so much. I feel that we all need to look after ourselves and stick up for ourselves with the medical profession, in honour of a man who saved many lives, mine included.

Chapter 14

Advice for our Partners and Families

A frequent cry of lament from desperate people with APS is that no one understands. Of course, for those not yet treated and still waiting to see a specialist it is a long rocky road with no one understanding them.

We can really feel desperately ill before treatment; it can feel as though there is no end to the agonies to go through. I know that before treatment I often felt like life wasn't worth living and only knowing I was loved and believed by those closest to me stopped me getting totally depressed.

Getting up every day and feeling ill every day is a soul-destroying experience. The importance of finding the right doctor and getting anticoagulation treatment cannot be stressed enough. It is not just that there is a danger of life threatening blood clots without treatment. Many of us suffered terribly both before and after diagnosis with terrifying symptoms for a long time before we finally received treatment. Sometimes that long drawn out limbo feels far worse than having a major crisis where everyone understands and takes care of you.

This is a serious problem for all of us with a long-term incurable illness, even after treatment most of us feel ill to some degree at some time each day, or if we feel well we usually get tired and grumpy at some point. It is never to the degree that we felt before treatment but since it is long-term, it is still life changing.

Energy which was once taken for granted must be rationed, jobs which once could be done any time, must be done first thing in the morning while we feel lively enough. Afternoon tasks which once were taken for granted are now obstacles to overcome or even impossible at times. Evenings can often be swallowed up snoozing in a chair when once you would have been out with friends.

Often partners are in denial about the seriousness of the problems facing us. Sometimes they can be plain and simply thoughtless, without meaning to be. They may accuse us of not pulling our weight or being lazy.

There are also those wonderful partners who read everything with you and want to understand and help as much as possible.

Most people's partners or family fall somewhere in between though. Some days they try very hard and are good, but at times they are so remote from your problems you feel alone and desperate.

This chapter is aimed at families and partners of those with APS and I hope, may ease a lot of pain and suffering.

How to live in harmony with us!

It can be done, honest!

The most longed-for need of an APS patient is for someone who will believe them.

It is bad enough feeling tired, aching all over, or feeling dizzy and muzzy-headed. It is damned near impossible to fight memory loss and forgetfulness.

The symptoms are very real and very hard to cope with at times. It is a nightmare at times getting doctors to listen and believe us, a disbelieving partner is really the last straw. If you can try to believe everything you are told by us, and never question it, or brush it off as nothing to worry about, it will be a huge help. It can be hard to see that your loved one is suffering, if they don't look ill, you may think they are faking it, but never, ever fall into that trap. Ask yourself, if she/he is faking this what are they getting out of it? I can tell you from experience...

nothing at all!

Usually all they get is to miss lots of things they really love doing.

Self Help?

Try to avoid all those self-help suggestions! Arrrgh! If I counted all the times someone has said, "If you lost weight, ate more fruit, took vitamins, took more exercise, took this miracle cure-all etc, perhaps you'll feel better!"

No, we will NOT feel better. We will feel patronised and belittled. If a cure were as simple as that don't you think we would have done it already?

Most people feeling ill really try to look after themselves, but would you want to go to the gym if every muscle and joint was aching already? Many of us feel as though we have been to the gym every day! The sad thing is that we haven't!

OK so losing weight is always a good idea, but if you feel worn out and ill it can be hard not to allow yourself a treat to cheer yourself up. Once we are taking Warfarin we can't get drunk anymore! It is one thing to deny yourself when you have a full and active life and feel great, but if you don't, it is just one more thing to worry about.

A good partner should try to encourage you if you really want to try to lose weight and exercise more but know that harping on about it all the time is just counterproductive and very upsetting when all you really want is to sleep a while!

Don't give in

Another gripe is that people say, "You mustn't give up." or "You'll really have to buck your ideas up!" Oh please! It is so easy to think that all we need is a good kick up the behind and we'll be fine. We have a blood-clotting problem, we have tested positive and our condition causes many diverse and upsetting symptoms, not least of all that it can kill us or leave us disabled unless we are correctly treated. How exactly are we to buck our ideas up?

It just isn't possible to be better by thought alone in this case. Although I find a positive attitude when it can be managed is a huge help.

I've got that as well

When people say, "Oh I have that happen to me" when you are trying to describe a symptom such as forgetfulness. Perhaps you do but not all the time.

You don't forget something you did half an hour ago; completely and utterly forget it with no chance of ever finding that memory again.

It is unnerving when that happens, it is not normal, it makes you feel afraid and a little sick, and unless you have a problem too, or are very elderly, it does not happen to you! Suggesting that you know how we feel is not true.

It is hurtful that you think that our problem is just a common one, and "nothing to get worked up about." It is usually affecting our lives badly and that needs acknowledgement, not dismissal.

Why don't you get up and go out?

It will cheer you up they say.

If your partner seems reluctant to join you on a trip out or an evening at the pub it is not just to be awkward or spoil your fun.

They may be tired or just not feel confident enough to face a crowded bar or restaurant. They are probably afraid that people will make a fuss should they say they feel unwell in public. Most of us will put on a brave front to please a partner or to avoid a confrontation. Try to talk together about trips out, think of the practical things (will there be somewhere to sit or rest) acknowledge that your partner may be feeling a little worried about whether they can cope. It is sometimes a scary business being out and about, compared to the relative safety and comfort of home.

I like to know that there is somewhere I can sit down if I need to and that my husband will listen if I say I've had enough. Armed with that knowledge I am willing to try most things, sometimes I surprise myself and I'm always glad I pushed myself a little.

Illness shouldn't mean sitting at home feeling sorry for yourself necessarily. All that is needed to have confidence in going out, is to know your companion understands, and will see that you get a seat if you need one and will take you home if you really need to go. These are little things, which make a big difference.

I can see that this chapter sounds negative, but I hear so many tales of desperately unhappy people who are on the verge of giving up through a simple lack of understanding.

Just take my word for it, I need a rest

Really all they need is someone to believe them unconditionally and not expect miracles from them. Someone who loves them and accepts that at times they are not smiley, happy people, even though they may desperately try to be. Someone who knows that the nasty words that were said when you were tired should be forgotten. Nasty words, temper flares and slammed doors should be calmly dealt with and soon forgotten, and the person concerned told to rest a while. I always find that a few quiet tears on my own when I'm tired and fed up and a sleep alters my mood magically!

What is needed is someone to say, "Ok you're bad tempered today, are you tired?" and if you say yes to that, they say "Go to bed for a while, leave what you're doing."

Have you ever felt exhausted?

Try to remember the last time you felt tired, after a sleepless night, perhaps with a sick child, or when you were ill yourself. It was overwhelming, all you wanted to do was sleep and you could think of nothing else; it was torture to have to keep going.

Now imagine feeling that tired several times a week, imagine that tiredness stopping you from doing things that you love or really need to get done, then imagine this is going to happen to you for the rest of your life. On top of that perhaps all your muscles ache or your head feels full of cotton wool, your toes keep getting sharp painful pins and needles, or go numb suddenly. Simple tasks, which you once did without a thought, are now major expeditions to be planned and worried over.

Would you get miserable at times? Wouldn't anyone? It would be abnormal not to!

Sometimes it is all in the mind literally!

It is useful if when your partner can't remember or gets lost in the middle of a sentence you can automatically prompt them to remember, especially when you are out with friends and forgetting things can be so embarrassing. Also, reminders to write notes in a diary or on a calendar will help. I also tick my diary when I take my tablets, as I have been known to forget whether I took them or not. That feels frustrating, as you think that if you really concentrate, you will remember but you just can't, however hard you try. It feels, as if there is nothing there to retrieve, the memory of that moment is gone forever.

Mobile phone calendars and reminders are a godsend. It saves me from forgetting where I should be so many times.

I ache all over

Aches and pains are common and uncomfortable, but hard to treat. The muscular pain we have may not be life threatening, but it can wear you down. It becomes hard to rest without constant aches and pains interfering. Joint pain is also a nuisance and when it's in the hips, finding a comfy position can be hard.

A little help is worth a lot of sympathy and running a hot bath or getting an electric blanket for the bed is helpful. If your partner is warm, then pains will seem less troublesome and knowing you care is half the battle.

We need someone who is on our side

Hospital visits are awful when you're alone. I know it's not practical to trail your partner around every clinic but if you can go to just the important ones, you can hear the truth about your loved one's condition from a doctor and hopefully get a better understanding of it. Also, now and then there may be bad experiences with less helpful doctors (I hope, as time goes by this will happen less and less), and a backup from you about the severity of symptoms can be really needed.

Don't spoil the good times

It isn't all doom and gloom. There will be lots of times when your partner feels well and fine. There will be times that they want to burn the midnight oil, go dancing, have some fun and you may think to yourself perhaps, "there's nothing really wrong with them". They may manage a long day out without showing any signs of illness or even have a week of feeling well and seem full of life.

Don't spoil a snatched moment of really enjoying life by saying, "Huh! I thought you were meant to be ill." We are ill! There are times when we can forget that though and times when we feel quite well for a few days or even weeks. It is good that we can have that time; it reminds us that good times aren't over, and life is worth living really. We may be exhausted the next day, but a good night out can be worth a rough day tomorrow.

A week of good days will be remembered for a long time and become treasured memories, if they are really enjoyed to the full.

I will never forget a holiday I had where I was lucky and felt just like the old me. I really enjoyed myself and walked all over. I even climbed some rocks to the top of a waterfall without feeling tired or ill at all. Even if that never came again I will always remember that holiday fondly (I do feel quite sure I will get another week like that though!). I don't think I could have enjoyed it as much if I was being constantly reminded that I was meant to be ill! All I heard was an occasional "are you alright?" that was appreciated, and I was thrilled to be able to keep saying, "Yes thanks!"

But all you talk about is APS

Sometimes it may feel as if all your once active and fun-loving partner wants to do is talk about their illness. It is hard not to when you are living with it every day. We can forget that our partners have things to talk about and troubles of their own. It may seem very selfish of us but rather than getting annoyed and saying, "All I ever hear about is APS!" Try to be a little gentler. Suggest that though you will listen once a day to all their troubles if they need it, but sometimes there are other things to talk about as well.

Try to discuss that suggestion at a quiet moment when your partner is not stressed or tired out. It can be hard to be reasonable when you feel hard done to.

Perhaps if it were you in their shoes you would be getting a little obsessed at times, try to be kind if you can.

Don't give me your stress

Stress makes all illness worse especially autoimmune illnesses. If you are fit and well, you can cope with stress. If you have Hughes Syndrome stress can literally cause a flare up of symptoms, which can lead to more serious problems. When we are subjected to stress it can be felt as physical symptoms which lead to physical illness. Try to protect us from stressful situations where possible.

Support groups are no substitute. Support groups are all well and good, but if the ones you love refuse to understand, a support group is a poor substitute.

I find that the APS patient who is most able to cope and least likely to be depressed is one with a helpful partner and family.

If you were ill wouldn't you want this? Wouldn't anyone?

Chapter 15

Travelling and APS

Travelling can be a little daunting for anyone with an illness of any sort.

Some people choose not to travel by air due to the risk from blood clots, others think nothing of it, but it is down to how you feel about the prospect.

For those who do love to travel whether it is by air, land or sea I have compiled a list of useful tips and ideas.

Most of these have come from my friends on the Delphi APS forum. This forum was popular in the early 2000s, before Facebook. Mark, who set up the forum, was a seasoned traveller so these are, in the main, his suggestions.

1) Be sure to wear your Medic Alert bracelet/necklace always.

2) Keep a list of your tablets and doses, for example: Warfarin 10mg once a day. Keep the list in a couple of places. One list can be in your luggage and one in your wallet or with your passport. If you and your medicines get separated at least you will have a list to take to a doctor or pharmacy. Your doctor may be able to print you a list off if you ask him/her.

3) You may get questioned about your tablets at Customs. It is a good idea to ensure they are all in original containers with your doctor's name on it. Your pharmacy may be able to label up smaller tablet bottles, to hold a weeks' worth of tablets instead of having to take a month's supply with you! It is always best to take enough though, in case of delays, a spare day or two's tablets can be useful.

4) Ensure that you are covered by health/travel insurance. Make a special point of checking you are covered for this illness and any others you may have. I would simply not bother going unless a good insurance was in place.

5) Check with your doctor that it is ok to travel, in plenty of time.

6) On planes try to get an aisle seat or an exit row so there is room to move your legs about and it is easy to get up and walk about. Mention that you have a blood clotting illness if it helps you get a good seat. Do as much as you can to keep your blood on the move. Go to the lavatory a few times, stretch, wear the specially designed "flight socks" to help the blood back out of your legs.

7) This may not be very popular, but don't drink alcohol and fly! You are already getting less oxygen at altitude, alcohol only complicates things.

8) Try not to push yourself too hard. Leave yourself plenty of time for everything. Arrive at the airport early and take things slowly. It is better to be bored for a while waiting, than exhausted by all the running between gates.

9) If you are travelling to a country with dubious medical services, find out before you go, where the British/US/Australian etc Embassy is. Imagine how hard it is to explain APS to the average English-speaking doctor. Now imagine it in a foreign language, it doesn't bear thinking about!
In fact, even if the medical care is wonderful in the country you are travelling to, if you don't speak the language, someone from the Embassy could be a lifesaver.
Also find out how to say Antiphospholipid Syndrome and Warfarin, in the language of the country you are visiting if it is at all possible! It could be useful!

10) If travelling alone, be sure that friends/relatives know your itinerary and have phone numbers to contact you. Perhaps you could ring them at a set time each day, so they know you are ok. I will repeat for lone travellers NEVER, EVER remove your Medic Alert bracelet. It could be the only way that anyone knows what is wrong with you if you have an accident.

11) If you have any old illnesses that may reoccur then be sure to take some medication for that complaint with you. If you have it, you won't need it but if you don't...

12) If airport security should look at your tablets, then stay calm. Be sure that the tablets get put back in the correct containers. You have nothing to hide, so don't panic about it; it is only a routine.

Ask for a seat if they take a long time and you feel tired. Always put medication in hand luggage in case your suitcase gets mislaid.

13) Bear in mind that the idea of moving about isn't just for air travel but also for any long journey. Wriggle your toes, stand up and walk if possible, or if in a car, stop and have a coffee and stretch your legs.

14) I always carry a copy of Prof Hughes patient's book in my handbag. I feel safer if any doctor treating me can read that first. It just backs up what you are trying to tell them if you have any problems. In these internet days a couple of websites stored on your smart phone may be easier.

15) Once you've done all these things, try to relax and enjoy yourself. All we can ever do is the best we can. Our lives will always have risky moments; everyone's has an element of risk. It does seem that we have a bit more to worry over though doesn't it!

Oh well, sit back, enjoy the view and forget your cares. Reality will be back soon enough! Have a great holiday!

Chapter 16

Graham Hughes International Charity and other sources of support

In 2017 many long-time patients who had supported the Hughes Syndrome Foundation ever since it started at St Thomas' hospital were dismayed to hear that the trustees had decided to change the name to APS Support UK. We were upset as Prof Hughes was the person who discovered the illness back in the early 1980s and worked on it with his team until he came up with the tests and a full description of the illness in 1983.

There is only one Graham Hughes and he has saved so many lives worldwide, trained so many doctors, done so much research and most importantly listened to and helped his patients. He works hard to spread awareness and is respected by those in his field.

This man has made people in wheelchairs walk again, even the blind see again. This is not just one-off situations either, it is routine for him.

Many of us were heart broken that the charity we considered our own was dropping his name.

Professor Graham Hughes is not just my doctor, he is my friend.

For him now to have his name removed from the charity he set up with Hilary Clark was unbelievable to many people.

In any case the decision was made, and a group of patients and friends rallied around and helped to set up GHIC. This charity is an international one and deals with both awareness of Hughes Syndrome and Lupus.

Thanks must go to those who set it up and those who helped with funding or their time.

It was launched in 2017 and the website is a mine of information.

APS Support UK is still a good website for information and awareness, indeed I would recommend it. There can never be too much information online for patients to read and educate themselves.

However, GHIC will be running patient's days in London and has the support of 78 medical experts as an advisory committee, also it is the only charity with our dear Prof Hughes involved. If we can't be grateful to the man who has done so much, so selflessly for all of us then who can we be grateful to? Thank you, Professor Graham Hughes, a very special man.

Support Groups

The main support groups for the illness that I know of are on Facebook. Most of them were set up by an amazing woman Hazel Edwards. She puts others in front of herself even though she is often extremely ill herself. She has a great team of patients helping her and her groups are a source of comfort and information for people worldwide.

Mary Foord-Brown and Lynne Diggins run a support group on Health Unlocked which is highly thought of and has helped so many frightened newbies to this illness with kind advice.

All these ladies have worked tirelessly to spread awareness and support others whilst dealing with their own illnesses and have voluntarily given their time to do this.

Charities are a great thing to raise awareness and share information and support groups are a lifeline to patients. Also don't forget that as well as my books, Professor Hughes has written many, as have his colleagues.

May you all get the help you need.

A final note: This book is written from my own and other's experiences of Antiphospholipid or Hughes Syndrome. It is intended to work as if it was a good and knowledgeable friend you can turn to for sensible and easy to understand answers to the many questions you have. It is not a medical book and I am not medically trained. In no way should this book be used in place of your doctor at any time. It is full of my personal opinions and information, which I believe to be true from my own research and speaking to other APS patients. That knowledge is no substitute for proper medical help and I would never suggest it was.